Fit Babe Energy

Transform Your Body, Reclaim Your Confidence, Find Your Fearless over 40

By: Chrissy Gray

Dedication

To my three incredible sons, who keep me on my toes and inspire me every single day. You each bring your own unique spark to this world—so different, yet so brilliantly creative. I pray you continue to shine like the precious, one-of-a-kind gems God made you to be.

With all my love,

Mom

Table of Contents

Introduction

From Invisible to Invincible

For most of my life, I mastered one thing: being invisible. No, I'm not talking about some superhero power. I'm talking about blending into the background, ducking out of photos, and praying no one would notice me. I was the queen of small talk, the expert at staying quiet, and the absolute champ of making sure no one had to pay attention to me.

But here's the thing about being invisible—it catches up with you. One day, while scrolling through Facebook, I decided to send a friend request to someone I went to school with for years. We shared classrooms, the same lunch tables, and even went to the same church. I figured he'd remember me. Easy, right? Wrong.

When his response popped up, it was like a gut punch: "My memory is blank. Remind me how I know you?" Ouch.

In that moment, I realized just how small I'd made myself. I had spent so much time blending in that I had practically disappeared. And you know what? That wasn't just some Facebook glitch. That was my life.

The Wake-Up Call I Didn't Know I Needed

Sure, that Facebook message hurt. But it also woke me up. It made me realize just how much of my life I had spent fading into the background, letting self-doubt call the shots. That was the moment I decided something had to change. I wasn't going to live life hiding anymore. I wasn't going to let myself be invisible, not to the world, and most importantly, not to myself.

And if you're reading this, I'm guessing you've had your own wake-up call. Maybe you've felt stuck, overlooked, or like life is happening to everyone but you. I get it. I've been there.

Why the World Needs to See You

The fact that you're holding this book right now tells me one thing—you're ready. You're ready to stop hiding, to stop doubting yourself, and to start living a life that's fully yours. And here's what I've learned: the world needs to see you. Yes, you. Not some filtered, edited version of you. The real, brilliant, messy, powerful you.

You're not here to fade into the background. You're here to take up space, to shine, and to show the world what you're capable of. Trust me, the moment you start showing up for yourself, the world will start showing up for you too.

Attracting the Life You Deserve

Once you stop hiding, everything changes. It's not some woo-woo magic—it's science. When you start believing in yourself and owning your space, you attract the life you've always wanted. Opportunities appear, relationships flourish, and life just starts to align.

Does it happen overnight? Nope. Will it be easy? Also, nope. But I'll tell you this: it will be worth it.

Confidence Isn't Perfection

Here's something I want you to remember: confidence isn't about being perfect. It's about showing up, flaws and all, and saying, "Here I am." It's about keeping the promises you make to yourself, even when it's hard. It's about knowing you deserve to be seen, to be heard, and to be valued.

If I can go from feeling invisible to feeling invincible, I know you can too.

Let's Get Started

So, are you ready? Ready to stop playing small and start living big? This journey isn't just about transforming your body—it's about transforming the way you see yourself. It's about embracing your Fit Babe Energy—the energy that will take you from feeling invisible to unstoppable.

The world is ready to meet the real you. Now, it's time for you to meet her too. Let's GO!

Chapter 1

The Day My Body Broke
(Or So I Thought)

Let me paint you a picture. I was 39, pregnant with my third son, and my body felt like it had thrown in the towel. Not just a gentle wave of surrender, but a full-blown white flag flapping in the wind, signaling total defeat. My body, it seemed, had gone AWOL.

Now, I should rewind a bit. Once upon a time, I was *that* skinny girl. The one who had a foolproof (though incredibly unhealthy) way of dropping weight—just stop eating. It worked like a charm in my 20s. Anytime life felt out of control, I'd control the one thing I could: what went in my mouth, or more specifically, what *didn't* go in my mouth. I could "fix" anything with a little starvation. Oh, the joys of youthful ignorance.

Fast forward to my 40s, and it was like my body flipped me off. The old tricks? They didn't just stop working—they rebelled. I breastfed my third baby, expecting to shed pounds like my friends who claimed breastfeeding was the golden ticket to weight loss. Instead, I gained weight. It was as if my body decided it was preparing for the apocalypse, hoarding fat like it was preparing for a long winter's nap.

A Tampon and a Bladder That Checked Out

Just when I thought I had a handle on the whole "pregnancy body changes" thing, my bladder decided to give me the middle finger. Enter posterior vaginal prolapse, aka rectocele, which hit me after my first son's birth. Thanks, childbirth! My body was essentially saying, "We're done here," and my bladder? It tapped out.

Here's the part no one talks about: I relied on a *super tampon*. Not for the usual reasons, mind you, but to literally hold my bladder in place. Yeah, you read that right. A tampon became my body's structural support. There's nothing like walking around knowing a tampon is basically the only thing keeping your insides from throwing a party on the outside.

This wasn't just aging—it was a full-on betrayal. I felt like a patchwork quilt of tampons and willpower, holding myself together by sheer stubbornness. It was a surreal, disheartening moment to realize that my body, the one I thought I had some control over, had essentially thrown in the towel.

Diastasis Recti: The Gap That Kept On Giving

The real kicker, though, was something I had never even heard of: diastasis recti. That's a fancy term for when your abdominal muscles decide to go their separate ways—permanently. My doctor looked at me and said, "Oh yeah, it's probably permanent. You'll never be able to do ab exercises again."

Wait, what? Never again? My brain went into overdrive. Did she just say I was *permanently* broken?

Let me tell you, hearing those words felt like a gut punch—literally. And while my abs had physically separated, it felt like my entire identity had fractured along with them.

Accepting the New Normal (Or Not)

After that appointment, I stood in front of the mirror and stared at the stranger staring back. Was this it? Was this my "new normal"? Sagging skin, a bladder on life support, and a four-finger gap between my abs? There was a part of me that wanted to throw in the towel and accept my fate as this broken version of myself. But deep down, there was another part—an angrier part—that wasn't ready to give up.

Sure, my body felt like it had betrayed me, but I wasn't ready to believe that this was the end of the story. I refused to believe I was broken.

The Day Everything Changed

You know how people always talk about those life-changing moments where everything suddenly clicks into place? Well, I had one of those. It didn't come with a chorus of angels or a flash of light, though. It came in the form of sheer frustration and a refusal to give up on myself.

I realized something important: I wasn't broken. My body had been through three pregnancies, diastasis recti, and a prolapsed bladder. It had been through war. But that didn't mean I was defeated. It just meant I needed a new strategy. A new way to move forward. Fit Babe Energy wasn't about a perfect body—it was about reclaiming the power I thought I had lost.

Fit Babe Energy: A Mindset Shift

Fit Babe Energy became my mantra. It wasn't just about fixing my abs or losing weight—it was about shifting my mindset. Every day that I showed up for myself, whether it was through a quick workout or simply swapping a less healthy habit for a better one, I was reinforcing that energy. And slowly, but surely, the results followed.

I wasn't just seeing changes in my body—my mind was transforming. I no longer felt like a victim of my circumstances or a passenger in my life. I was in control. And let me tell you, that feeling was better than any number on the scale.

Small Wins, Big Changes

The beauty of this journey was that it wasn't about the big, dramatic moments. It was the small wins that made the biggest difference. A 10-minute workout here, swapping out processed snacks for something better there—it all added up. Every small victory was a brick in the foundation of my new life.

And guess what? I didn't diet. I didn't starve. I didn't count a single calorie. I allowed myself to eat what I loved—yes, that includes pizza and fries. Fit Babe Energy wasn't about deprivation; it was about embracing life fully, loving myself fully, and building a body that supported the life I wanted to live.

A New Way Forward

Today, I'm 60 pounds lighter, but more importantly, I'm stronger—physically and mentally. I've transformed my body, yes, but more than that, I've transformed my entire life. I'm no longer just a tired mom of three—I'm stronger, healthier, and more vibrant than I've ever been.

And now? Now, I'm on a mission to share this energy with other women who feel like they're too far gone. Because here's the truth: you're not broken. You've still got so much left in you. Fit Babe Energy is how you tap into that power.

The Beginning of Something Bigger

If you've ever felt like your body has betrayed you—like you're too old, too tired, or too broken to start over—let me be the one to tell you: you're wrong. You are not broken. You are a powerhouse waiting to rise. And trust me, once you tap into that Fit Babe Energy, there's no stopping you.

This is just the beginning of your story, not the end. The best part? You get to write the next chapter.

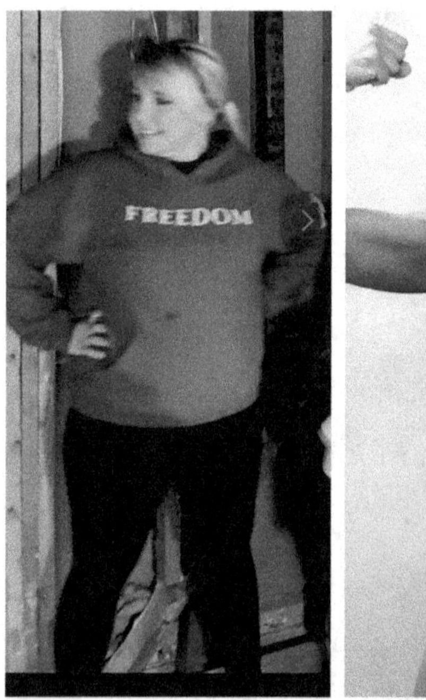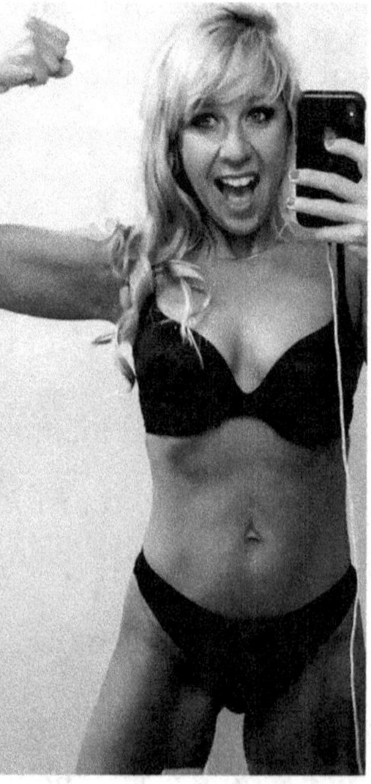

Here is a photo of me in 2022 and of me as of writing this book.

Chapter 2

My Epic (and Hilarious) Return
to the Gym

Let me start by saying that I had been a gym member for years. I had the card, the gym bag, the water bottle, and even a drawer full of workout clothes that I'd occasionally wear while lounging around the house. But here's the truth: I had never actually ventured into the weight room. Nope, I was a cardio queen. I'd walk right past the dumbbells, barbells, and the burly people lifting them, making a beeline for the elliptical machines and treadmills, where I could plug in my headphones, zone out, and pretend like I was doing something productive.

Why weights? They terrified me. The weight room was this intimidating land where people grunted, sweated profusely, and threw around heavy metal like it was nothing. Meanwhile, I couldn't even figure out how to adjust the seat on a leg press machine without feeling like an idiot. So, I stuck to what I knew—cardio. It was easy, safe, and didn't require me to ask for help or make a fool of myself. And it's not like cardio wasn't working. I mean, I was staying fit, kind of. But deep down, I knew I was avoiding the one thing that could really help me get stronger: the weights.

But one day, something shifted. I was tired of being intimidated. I was tired of looking at the weight room like it was some exclusive club I wasn't cool enough to join. So, I decided—no more hiding. It was time to face the weights. And let me tell you, what followed was nothing short of hilarious.

The Cardio Queen Turned Weight Room Novice

For years, I had been a loyal subject to the cardio machines. I'd climb on the elliptical, run on the treadmill, and occasionally attempt a spin class (and by attempt I mean look up at the board and keep walking). Cardio was comfortable. It didn't require much thought. You get on the machine, you press start, and boom—you're working out. Plus, there's something about mindlessly moving while listening to the *Taylor Swift RED album* that's oddly satisfying.

But while I was logging hours on the elliptical, something started gnawing at me. I wasn't really *seeing* the changes I wanted. Sure, I was starting to get active, but I wasn't feeling stronger or more confident. And let's be honest, cardio can only do so much. The weight room was where the magic happened, where people were building muscles, strength, and bodies that made them feel like superheroes.

So, I decided to step out of my comfort zone and into the unknown territory of the weight room. And let me tell you—it was like stepping onto another planet.

My First Day in the Weight Room: A Comedy of Errors

Imagine walking into a room filled with people who look like they've been lifting since birth, and then there's me—standing in the corner, clutching my water bottle like a lifeline. I walked in with zero clue what I was doing. In fact, my entire strategy was to look around and try to mimic what other people were doing. It wasn't the best plan, but hey, I figured it was better than standing there frozen in fear.

The first machine I attempted was the leg press. You'd think it would be simple. It's a chair with a big platform where you push with your legs—how hard could it be? Apparently, very hard, because I couldn't even figure out how to adjust the seat. I must have fiddled with the settings for a good five minutes, pretending like I was just "taking my time," while secretly praying no one was watching me.

Then came the dumbbells. Oh, the dumbbells. I picked up a pair of 10-pound weights and felt like I had just lifted a car. My arms shook like I was trying to bench press a refrigerator, and within seconds, I was ready to put them back down and call it a day. Meanwhile, people around me were throwing around weights like they were made of air, and here I was, struggling to lift what felt like the equivalent of a wet noodle.

I was embarrassed. I was sweating in places I didn't know could sweat. But I was determined not to quit. And that's when something amazing happened—I started to laugh.

Laughing Through the Struggle

You know what's funny about the weight room? Everyone is in their own world. I was so focused on what people might think of me that I didn't realize they weren't thinking about me at all. People were busy doing their own thing, working on their own goals. No one cared if I fumbled with the leg press or struggled to lift a dumbbell. It was all in my head.

So, I decided to let go of the fear of looking foolish and just embrace the fact that I was a beginner. And once I did that, the whole experience became so much more fun. I started laughing at myself—literally. I'd drop a weight, trip over a bench, and instead of getting embarrassed, I'd chuckle and move on. Because really, who cares? Everyone starts somewhere.

And here's the best part: after a few days, things started to click. I wasn't fumbling with the machines as much. I was getting the hang of the movements. And while I was still far from being the next powerlifting champion, I was making progress. And progress, no matter how small, felt incredible.

The Myth of the Weight Room Superhumans

One thing that had always kept me away from the weight room was this belief that I didn't belong. I thought it was a place reserved for people who already knew what they were doing, people who had been lifting for years and looked like Greek statues carved out of marble. But here's what I realized: the weight room isn't just for the seasoned pros—it's for everyone.

Sure, there are people who can bench press their body weight without breaking a sweat, but there are also people just like me—people who are learning, trying, and showing up. And that's all that really matters.

It doesn't matter how much you can lift or how perfect your form is. What matters is that you're there, putting in the effort, challenging yourself, and stepping outside of your comfort zone. That's where the real transformation happens.

Cardio vs. Weight Training: The Truth

Okay, let's address the elephant in the room—cardio. If you're anything like I was, you might be thinking, "But I need to do cardio to lose weight, right?" Wrong. Let me tell you a little secret: you don't have to spend hours on the treadmill to get in shape. In fact, weight training is one of the only and most effective ways to burn fat, build muscle, and transform your body over 40.

Cardio is great for your heart, don't get me wrong. And there's nothing wrong with throwing in a good run or a spin class every now and then. But if your goal is to build a strong, toned body, you need to lift weights. And don't worry, I'll go into more detail on why you won't have to rely on cardio to achieve your goals later in the book. (You don't have to be a slave to the treadmill!)

The Power of Showing Up

The hardest part of any fitness journey isn't the workout itself—it's showing up. Whether it's showing up to the gym for the first time, stepping into the weight room, or even just getting out of bed when you'd rather sleep in, showing up is half the battle. But here's the thing: the more you show up, the easier it gets.

That first day in the weight room was terrifying, but each day after that got a little less scary. The machines didn't seem so intimidating. The weights didn't feel so heavy. And the people? They were just people—doing their own thing, just like me.

The Real Strength: Overcoming Fear

Looking back, the biggest obstacle I had to overcome wasn't physical—it was mental. It wasn't the weights or the machines that were holding me back—it was my fear. Fear of looking foolish, fear of failing, fear of not being strong enough.

But here's the truth: the moment you face that fear, you realize how insignificant it really is. It's like shining a light in the dark and realizing the monster you were so afraid of was just a shadow. Once I stopped letting fear control me, I found strength I didn't know I had.

In Conclusion: Embrace the Journey

So, here's the takeaway from my first epic adventure into the weight room: it doesn't matter where you start, how much you can lift, or how awkward you feel. What matters is that you start. Step into that weight room, pick up those dumbbells, and give yourself permission to be a beginner.

And trust me, you don't have to be perfect. You don't have to lift the heaviest weights or master every machine right away. You just have to show up, put in the work, and keep moving forward. Because at the end of the day, that's what Fit Babe Energy is all about—showing up for yourself, even when it's hard, even when it's uncomfortable, and even when you don't have it all figured out.

So, if you're ready to step out of the cardio corner and into the world of weight training, take a deep breath, laugh at the awkwardness, and embrace the journey. You've got this.

Chapter 3

Intermittent Fasting, Saxony Whalen, and the Midlife Glow-Up I Didn't See Coming

Let's get one thing straight right off the bat: when I decided to change my life, I didn't do it by following some dramatic detox or signing up for a 5 a.m. boot camp in the park. Nope. I did what any reasonable person in their 40s does when they're tired of feeling like crap—I looked for an easier, smarter way to feel better without hating my life.

That's when I stumbled across what might just be the least aggressive diet hack ever: intermittent fasting. Now, before you roll your eyes and picture me sitting around sipping bone broth while chanting, let me explain. Intermittent fasting isn't a cult (I promise). It's just a really sneaky way to trick your body into thinking it's a fat-burning machine without cutting out all the things that make life worth living.

The Accidental Genius of Eating Once a Day

Here's how I found it: one day, while scrolling through Instagram—because that's where all life-changing ideas happen these days—I came across Dr. Mindy Pelz. She was the voice of reason on fasting, breaking it down in a way that finally made sense to me. And let me tell you, I was ready to hear someone explain how I could eat less without giving up food altogether. I mean, I love food. Not "Instagram avocado toast" food, but real food. Like pizza.

Dr. Pelz talked about how intermittent fasting helps with hormonal balance, especially for women over 40. And I was like, *Hold up, hormonal balance?* Because if you're over 40 and you've ever wanted to throw something (or someone) out the window for absolutely no reason, you know hormones are no joke.

Her approach was simple: for women in their 40s, intermittent fasting could do wonders for balancing insulin, improving energy levels, and—get this—burning fat. She wasn't only talking about your typical 16:8 fasting where you skip breakfast and eat lunch. No, she introduced me to OMAD—One Meal A Day, or as I like to call it, the "Get Your Life Back" plan.

It sounds extreme, right? Eating just one meal a day? But here's the wild part: it worked. For me, it meant fasting for about 20 hours and eating within a 4-hour window. The rest of the day, I could sip on black coffee, tea, or water, and then around dinnertime, I'd have my one glorious meal. I actually liked to start my eating window around 11 am and finish by 3 pm. And no, it wasn't just salad leaves. We're talking real food—protein, veggies, healthy fats—the stuff that fuels your body.

The Moment I Realized I Didn't Have to Obsess Over Food

The first few days of OMAD were... interesting. I won't lie; the idea of not eating for 20 hours day sounded like torture. But I quickly discovered something amazing: I wasn't as hungry as I thought I'd be. In fact, after the first week, I realized how much of my eating was out of boredom or habit rather than actual hunger.

With OMAD, I stopped obsessing over food. There were no more meal preps, no more endless snacking, and best of all—no more calorie counting. I wasn't living in constant fear of food anymore. It was like I had finally been given the freedom to *not think about eating* all the time, and that, my friends, was revolutionary.

Intermittent fasting, especially OMAD, wasn't just about shrinking my waistline (though that happened too, 15 pounds gone, thank you very much). It was about clarity. Mental clarity, physical clarity, and just a better understanding of what my body actually needed. It wasn't six small meals a day. Who knew?

Why OMAD is a Midlife Superpower

Here's something magical about OMAD when you're over 40: it gives you control over your body in a way you probably haven't felt in years. All those hormonal mood swings, bloating, and late-night carb cravings? OMAD helps tame them. When you give your

body a long stretch of fasting time, it finally has a chance to reset
and heal itself.

Women over 40 aren't just dealing with metabolism that's slowed
down like an old Windows computer—we're battling hormonal
chaos too. Insulin resistance, inflammation, cortisol spikes... all of it
works against us. But fasting helps balance all that. It gives your body
a break from constantly processing food, and in that downtime, it
works to repair, reset, and burn off that pesky fat you've been trying
to get rid of since your 30s.

It's like hitting a giant reset button on your body.

And trust me, fasting doesn't mean deprivation. It means
freedom. You get one big meal where you can eat satisfying, delicious
food without feeling like you're cheating on some impossible diet.
And you know what? You actually *enjoy* that meal more because
you're not stuffing your face mindlessly while watching Netflix.

Enter: Saxony Whalen—The Woman Who Blew My Mind (And Made Me Obsessed with Legs)

Now, intermittent fasting was going great, but there was
something missing. I was losing weight, sure, but I wasn't getting
stronger. Enter Saxony Whalen (married to Sean Whalen of Lions
Not Sheep). Let me paint you a picture: I'm scrolling through
Instagram, sipping my black coffee (thank you, OMAD), and I see
this woman. She's not just fit; she's strong. She's not some 22-year-
old fitness Barbie. She's a woman, like me, who's been through

some stuff. When I found her she was in her late 30s, had two kids, and her legs look like they could crush a watermelon.

And I was like, *Who is this Goddess?*

Sax was different from every other fitness influencer I'd seen. She wasn't slinging detox teas or posing next to a plate of kale. She was real. She was raw. And she was unapologetically powerful. This was the kind of energy I needed in my life.

The Instagram Rabbit Hole of Inspiration

I'll admit it: I became a little obsessed. Not in a creepy way, but in a *this-woman-is-living-the-life-I-want-to-be-living* kind of way. I deep-dived into her Instagram feed like I was conducting research for a PhD. Every picture, every caption, every podcast she and her husband posted (the Sean and Sax Show)—I soaked it all in.

What I loved about Sax was that she didn't pretend her life was perfect. She didn't act like getting fit and staying strong was some kind of fairytale journey. She had kids, responsibilities, and stretch marks. She wasn't pretending to be perfect—she was owning her imperfections, and that made her even more badass.

The Leg Inspiration That Launched a Thousand Squats

Let's talk about her legs for a minute. Those legs were the kind of legs you'd dream about having while doing a mind-numbing cardio session on the elliptical. They were strong, defined, and just... powerful. And I decided then and there that I wanted to have legs like that. Not because I wanted to be her, but because I wanted to feel as strong as she looked.

I saved about 4 pictures of her and added them to my favorites. I don't know if you remember but in the 90s it was common to buy a bikini and hang it on the fridge so everytime you walked by you'd see what you want to be and hopefully not overeat. Well every time I opened my photo album on my phone smack dab front and center were Sax's legs reminding me of what was possible.

But it wasn't just the legs. It was the whole package—her confidence, her strength, her willingness to show up every day and do the hard stuff. That's what I was after. Sax wasn't just my leg goal; she was my life goal. Relationship. Fitness. Mindset

More Than a Fitspo—She Was a Muse

Sax wasn't just another influencer to me. She became my muse. Her energy was contagious. She wasn't trying to sell perfection; she was showing the power of showing up. I didn't need to be a supermodel or run marathons to feel strong. I just needed to be consistent. I needed to tap into that Fit Babe Energy that Sax embodied so effortlessly.

Her message wasn't about achieving some perfect body. It was about becoming the best, strongest, most confident version of yourself. That resonated with me. I wasn't trying to be Sax—I was trying to be *me*, but stronger.

Fit Babe Energy: It's Not About Perfection

Here's what I realized watching Sax do her thing: Fit Babe Energy isn't about doing it all perfectly. It's not about never missing a workout or always eating clean. It's about showing up, doing your best, and owning your journey, no matter how messy it gets. Sax wasn't perfect, and she wasn't trying to be. She was just real, and that was more inspiring than any airbrushed fitness model could ever be.

I started embracing that same energy in my own life. I stopped trying to be perfect, and I started showing up. Day after day, I put in the work, and slowly but surely, I started to see the results. Not just in my body, but in my confidence. I was owning my journey, just like Sax had shown me. And let me tell you, there's no better feeling than realizing you've got your own back.

The Journey Isn't About Becoming Someone Else— It's About Owning Your Space

At the end of the day, Sax's influence wasn't about me trying to become her. It was about me realizing that I could become more of myself. I didn't need to fit into someone else's mold—I just needed to show up for myself, every single day, and claim my space in this world.

And that's the beauty of Fit Babe Energy. It's not about looking like someone else or achieving some idealized version of fitness. It's about becoming the strongest, most confident version of you. It's about showing up, doing the hard stuff, and realizing that you are capable of so much more than you ever thought possible.

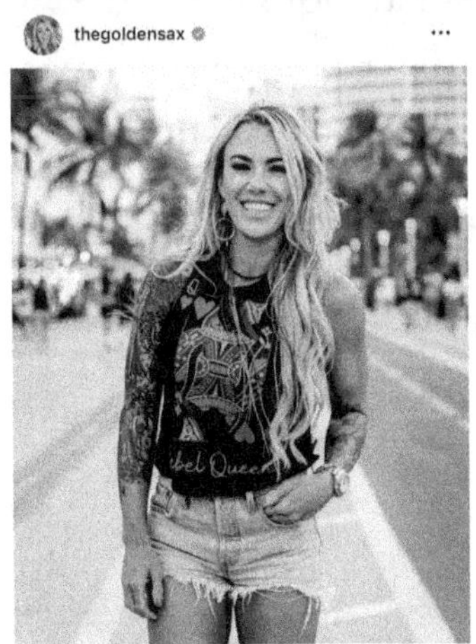

You can find Saxony on Instagram @thegoldensax

Chapter 4

The Trainer, The Transformation, and The No-Excuses Journey

Let's cut right to it. You're expecting me to tell you I hired a personal trainer after some deep soul-searching, right? Wrong. I didn't just hire *any* personal trainer. Nope, I went full-on diva and found the hottest trainer I could. Her name was Jillian, and let me tell you, her back and legs could probably start their own sports league. She was everything I needed: strong, badass, and—here's the kicker—she didn't take any of my excuses. None.

Jillian wasn't some fresh-faced fitness guru acting like life was a breeze. She had two kids, juggled everything like a boss, and still found time to deadlift her body weight. I mean, this woman was a machine. If one of her kids got sick? If they wanted to go away for a few days? No problem. She'd still find a way to get her workout in, killing it, while I'd be over here Googling, "Can you skip a workout because you have an ingrown toenail?" She made me figure it out, no whining allowed.

I sent her my daily workout journal like it was my personal diary—showing her every single thing I did. I didn't want to let her down. That accountability? It was gold. Jillian had me begging to stop more times than I'd care to admit, but guess what? She didn't let me quit. She knew my body could do more, even when I was ready to tap out. And she was right. Every single time.

Oh, and abs? Forget about it. She never gave me a single ab exercise, which, considering my diastasis recti, was a total relief. She told me the core would naturally get stronger without crunches, and you know what? She was 100% right. My diastasis recti eventually healed completely—without a single sit-up, hanging leg lift or crunch in sight. It was like she had a sixth sense for this stuff.

The Decision: Time to Get Serious

So, why did I decide to hire Jillian? Because I was done dabbling. Sure, I had lost some weight with intermittent fasting (thank you, OMAD), but I was tired of being the out of shape Mom who was pretty numb to file. I'd spent years doing the elliptical here and there, sort of like a yo-yo cardio queen, but I was scared—like, *terrified*—of the weightlifting area. You know the one. It's full of giant dudes grunting like they're in a lumberjack competition, and then there's me, trying not to make eye contact while pretending to be very interested in the water fountain or my shoe laces.

I had been a member of my gym for years and never ventured into the weight section until the month before. But enough was enough. It was time to face the fear. I didn't know what I was doing in the weight room. I wasn't just hiring Jillian because she had a killer physique—I hired her because she had the one thing I was lacking: killer confidence.

She was the type of trainer who didn't just get you fit—she made you realize you were capable of so much more than you ever thought. And that's what I needed. Someone to pull me out of my own head and say, "You've got this."

The First Jillian Workout: Reality Check

Let's talk about that first workout. I strolled into the gym feeling pretty good about myself. I mean, I'd been doing cardio for *years*. I had started venturing into the weight room. How hard could a workout with a trainer really be?

Two minutes in, I knew I was in over my head.

Jillian had me doing things I didn't even know were exercises. Bulgarian split squats? I thought she made those up just to mess with me. My legs were shaking so badly, I was sure I'd collapse right there on the floor. But Jillian? She was calm as ever. "You're doing great," she said, which I assumed was code for, "You look like you're dying, but I'm not going to tell you that because I want you to keep going."

And I did. Somehow, I kept going.

Here's the thing about weight training: it humbles you fast. All those years of cardio? Yeah, they didn't prepare me for this. My muscles were screaming, my heart was pounding, and I was pretty sure my face had turned an alarming shade of red. But there was something magical about it. After a few weeks and with every rep, every set, I could feel myself getting stronger. Not just physically, but mentally. Jillian had a way of pushing me just past the point where I thought I'd break. On leg day, my legs turned to jello by the time we finished. And every time, I came out the other side feeling like I could conquer the world.

No Excuses: Jillian's Way or No Way

The thing about Jillian was she didn't let me off the hook. Ever. I once tried to cancel a workout because one of my kids was sick. I thought it was a pretty good excuse, honestly. But Jillian? She wasn't having it. "You'll figure it out, I'll see you at 8," she said, completely unfazed by my crisis. And you know what? I did figure it out. Because when someone holds you accountable like that, you realize you're capable of a lot more than you give yourself credit for.

And that's the magic of a great trainer. Jillian wasn't there to coddle me or let me slide when things got hard. She was there to make sure I showed up for myself. No excuses, no drama, just results. And it worked. I found myself looking forward to our sessions, not just because I was getting stronger, but because I didn't want to let her down.

The Core Conundrum: Healing Without Abs

Here's where Jillian really blew my mind. After having three kids, my abs were shot. After all, I had diastasis recti. It left me with a four-finger gap between my abs, and every doctor I talked to said I'd need surgery to fix it.

But Jillian had other ideas. "We're not doing abs," she said during our first session. I thought she was joking. I mean, who hires a trainer and doesn't do ab work? But she was dead serious. "Your core will get stronger through the work we're doing," she explained. "We don't need to target it directly and make it worse."

I was skeptical, to say the least. I had always been told that crunches, sit ups, and hanging leg lifts were the holy grail of core strength. But Jillian had me doing everything *but* abs. Squats, RDLs, lunges, rows—you name it. And the weirdest thing happened: my core started getting stronger.

I wasn't doing any traditional ab exercises, but somehow, my diastasis recti started healing. I went from a four-finger gap to almost no gap at all. Without a single crunch. Jillian had been right all along. By strengthening the muscles around my core, the core itself got stronger too. It was like a fitness miracle.

The Accountability Factor: Why I Couldn't Quit

I kept a workout journal—like a fitness diary where I logged everything Jillian had me do. And let me tell you, there were days when I wanted to lie about my workouts. You know, just tweak the truth a little. "Oh yeah, totally did 4 sets of squats," when in reality I'd done three sets before deciding I was too tired.

But I couldn't lie to Jillian. There was something about her that made me want to be honest, even when I didn't want to. She'd check in with me regularly, and I didn't want to let her down. It wasn't even about the results at that point—it was about keeping my word. And that accountability was a game-changer.

When you've got someone in your corner, pushing you, expecting you to show up, it changes the whole game. You're not just doing it for yourself anymore—you're doing it because someone else believes in you, even when you don't believe in yourself.

No Magic Fix—Just Hard Work

Here's the thing no one tells you about personal trainers: they don't have magic wands. There's no secret formula that makes everything easier. It's still hard work. It's still showing up, day after day, and pushing yourself beyond what you thought you were capable of.

But that's the beauty of it. Jillian didn't promise me quick results. She didn't tell me I'd have abs of steel in six weeks or that I'd be able to deadlift a car by Christmas. What she did promise was that if I put in the work, I'd see the results. And she was right.

It wasn't overnight. There were days when I felt like I wasn't making any progress at all. But slowly, surely, the changes started happening. My body got stronger. My core healed. My confidence grew. And most importantly, I learned that I was capable of so much more than I ever thought.

The Unexpected Side Effect: Confidence

What I didn't expect when I hired Jillian was how much my mindset would shift. I thought I was hiring her to help me get physically stronger, and she did. But what she also did—without me realizing it—was build my confidence. With every rep, every set, I was proving to myself that I could do hard things. That I was stronger than my doubts, my fears, and my excuses.

That confidence? It spilled over into every area of my life. I found myself walking into rooms with a whole new level of confidence. I wasn't just the woman who was terrified of the weight room anymore—I was the woman who owned her space, in and out of the gym. And it wasn't just about the physical strength. It was about knowing I could push through the hard things, knowing I could show up for myself even when I didn't want to, and knowing that I had the power to make real, lasting changes in my life.

The Transformation Beyond the Gym

Here's the part nobody tells you: the work you put in at the gym doesn't just change your body—it changes your entire life. I found myself tackling challenges at work with more confidence, being more present with my kids, and setting boundaries where I needed to. I wasn't waiting for validation from anyone else anymore. I had proven to myself that I could follow through, that I could keep promises to myself, and that I could push past my own limitations.

And that's the real power of hiring a personal trainer like Jillian. It's not just about lifting weights or following a fitness plan—it's about becoming the strongest version of yourself, mentally and emotionally, as well as physically. It's about realizing that the only limits you have are the ones you've put on yourself.

No More Excuses, Just Results

When you've got someone like Jillian in your corner, you don't get to make excuses anymore. There's no "I'm too tired" or "I don't have time." Because Jillian wouldn't let me off the hook, I stopped letting myself off the hook. I stopped telling myself the story that I was too busy, too old, or that my body was just too fucked up to do anything about. Instead, I started showing up, every day, and doing the work.

And guess what? The results came. Slowly, yes. But they came. My body got stronger, my diastasis recti slowly healed, and my confidence soared. But more importantly, I learned that I was capable of so much more than I ever gave myself credit for. I stopped doubting myself and started trusting in the process, in the work, and in the fact that I was worthy of the effort.

The Power of Hiring the Right Trainer

Let me be clear: not all personal trainers are created equal. Hiring Jillian wasn't just about finding someone who could show me how to lift weights. It was about finding someone who would push me, hold me accountable, and not let me give up on myself. She wasn't there to coddle me or let me off the hook when things got tough—she was there to remind me that I was capable of more.

And that's the key to finding the right trainer. It's not about hiring someone who will make things easy for you—it's about hiring someone who will push you to be better, who will hold you accountable when you want to quit, and who will help you realize your full potential.

Jillian didn't just change my body. She changed my mindset, my confidence, and the way I approach challenges in every area of my life. She taught me that strength isn't just physical—it's mental, emotional, and it's built through showing up for yourself, day after day, even when it's hard.

The Bottom Line: Show Up, Do the Work

At the end of the day, the lesson I learned from Jillian was simple: show up, do the work, and trust the process. There's no magic formula, no quick fix, no easy way out. It's about putting in the effort, day after day, and trusting that the results will come.

And they do. Not overnight, not in some dramatic before-and-after transformation, but slowly, steadily, in ways you might not even notice at first. But one day, you'll look back and realize that you're not the same person you were when you started. You're stronger, more confident, and more capable than you ever thought possible.

So, if you're on the fence about hiring a personal trainer, let me just say this: do it. But don't just hire anyone. Find someone who will push you, hold you accountable, and believe in you even when you don't believe in yourself. Find your Jillian.

Because the real transformation isn't just in the weights you lift or the inches you lose—it's in the belief that you are worth the effort. And that belief? It changes everything.

In Conclusion: You're Stronger Than You Think

So here's what I want you to take away from this chapter: you are stronger than you think. Whether you've been scared to walk into the weight room, afraid to push yourself, or doubting whether you can really make a change—it's time to let that go.

You're capable of more than you've ever given yourself credit for. You just need to show up, do the work, and trust the process. And if you need a Jillian in your corner, don't be afraid to find her. Because having someone who believes in you, pushes you, and holds you accountable? It makes all the difference.

And remember: this isn't just about your body. It's about your mindset, your confidence, and your ability to tackle whatever life throws your way. So stop making excuses. Stop doubting yourself. And start showing up. Because once you do? There's no limit to what you can achieve.

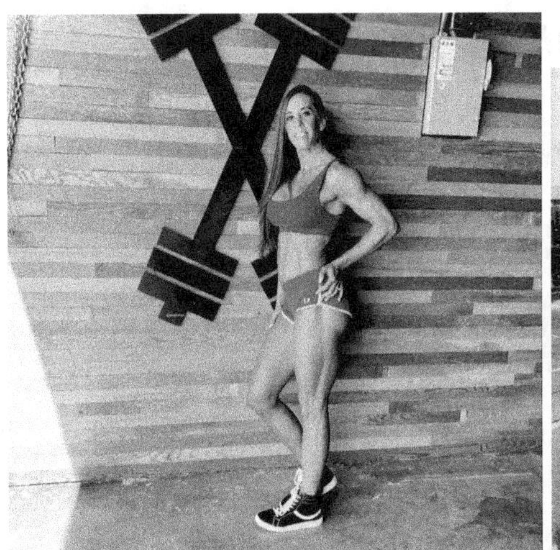

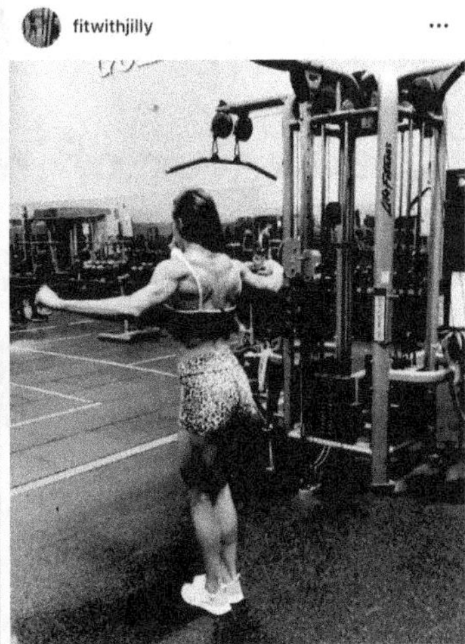

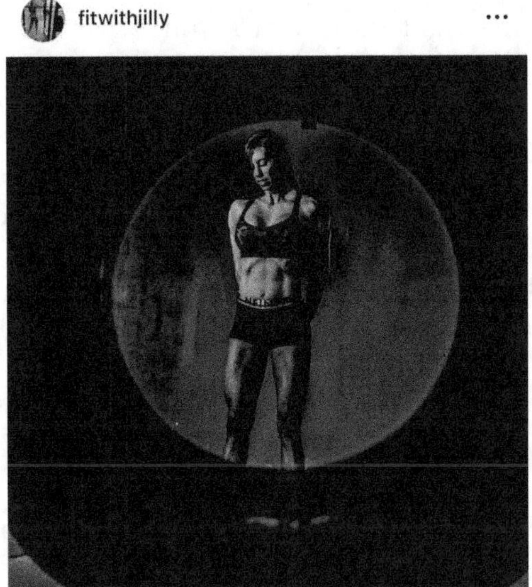

You can find Jillian on Instagram @fitwithjilly

Chapter 5

The Power of Makeup and the Magic of Confidence

Let me take you back to a moment in my life where everything changed—no, it wasn't in a gym or during one of those "rock bottom to breakthrough" moments you read about in fitness memoirs. Nope, my big shift happened in the most mundane of places: my bathroom, in front of the mirror, armed with the most unassuming weapon of all—makeup.

I know, sounds a little dramatic, right? But trust me, the shift was real. For years, I thought makeup was reserved for special occasions or for covering up some supposed "imperfection." But one day, something clicked. I started getting up a little earlier in the morning, applied just a touch of makeup, and suddenly, the woman staring back at me was someone I actually recognized. It wasn't about "hiding" or covering anything up—it was about enhancing what was already there. And with that, my confidence started to grow.

So yes, in a way, makeup became a game changer for me, but it wasn't just about looking good. It was about stepping into my own power and showing up for myself in ways I hadn't before. This, my friends, is where the story of makeup, confidence, and Fit Babe Energy truly begins.

Look Good, Feel Good, Do Good

For the last 13 years, *we've* been on a mission to help other women experience this same shift in confidence. Through **Sweet Minerals**—the makeup company my partners and I co-founded— we've spent over a decade empowering women to **look good, feel good, and do good**.

Now, I know that might sound like a catchy slogan (and it is), but it's also rooted in something much deeper. When you take care of your appearance, when you enhance your natural beauty in a way that makes you feel good about yourself, it changes everything. And I'm not just talking about how you look in selfies; I'm talking about how you show up in life.

As a team, we've built **Sweet Minerals** around a simple but powerful motto:

Look Good, Feel Good, Do Good.

When you feel good about how you look, you radiate that confidence into the world, which leads to positive actions and energy. Here's how it breaks down:

- **Look Good:** Makeup isn't about changing who you are. It's about accentuating the features you love and feeling good in your own skin. It's a tool for self-expression, creativity, and, ultimately, self-confidence.

- **Feel Good:** When you feel confident, it shows in everything you do. Whether you're heading into a meeting, running errands, or just going about your day, that inner glow radiates outward.

- **Do Good:** Here's where the magic happens—when you feel good, you're more likely to spread that positivity. You start showing kindness, lifting others up, and engaging in ways that create a ripple effect of good energy.

The Flawless Face and the Day I Finally Saw Myself Again

There was one day that stands out as the moment I realized how much power makeup had given me—and no, I wasn't in full glam or getting ready for some red-carpet event. It was just a regular day, and I was using our signature Sweet Minerals collection, the **Flawless Face.**

Now, if you're not familiar with the Flawless Face, let me paint a picture for you. This isn't the kind of makeup you layer on like a mask. It's designed to enhance your God-given beauty—giving your skin a radiant, healthy glow without making you feel like you're hiding behind a layer of foundation.

And when I first saw myself in the mirror after applying it, I had a powerful moment of recognition: "Wow, there I am."

I hadn't felt like "me" in a long time. Years of stress, raising kids, and feeling disconnected from my body had taken a toll. But in that moment, looking at my reflection, I saw the version of myself that I had forgotten was there all along.

The Rose-Colored Glasses and Teenage Heartbreak

Now, let's rewind a bit to my teenage years. You know that blissful age when you're naive, idealistic, and still wearing those metaphorical rose-colored glasses? Yep, that was me. I went to a private Christian school, sheltered from a lot of what was happening in the world, and held on to my innocence probably longer than most.

And like many girls my age, I fell in love—or at least, I thought I did. This tall, skinny 17-year-old boy came into my life, said all the right things, and before I knew it, I was convinced I had found the one. In my 15-year-old head, I was already planning our future. I mean, who doesn't fall madly in love at 15 and start picking out china patterns, right?

Spoiler alert: he broke my heart. We didn't get married, no happily ever after. Instead, my heart was shattered into a million pieces, and I spent the next few months listening to sad music, staring out of windows like I was in some kind of teenage soap opera. Looking back, it's hilarious. At the time, though? Oh, it was devastating.

Fast Forward 27 Years: The Ultimate Redemption

Now, let's jump ahead 27 years. Here I am, age 42, juggling businesses, raising kids, and feeling stronger in my skin than I ever had before. And wouldn't you know it? I run into him—the very same guy who broke my heart at 15.

And here's where things get interesting. I was telling him about Sweet Minerals, how we make the most amazing makeup on the planet, that it makes every woman's skin look flawless. I went on and on. And then, out of the blue, he says, "I see that. You look amazing."

Boom. 27 years of heartbreak and teenage angst erased in an instant. It felt like all those feelings of inadequacy, all those tears I shed over a boy who didn't even matter anymore, vanished with that one sentence. My confidence? Through the roof.

Now, let's be honest. What girl *doesn't* want her high school crush to tell her she looks amazing over the age of 40? I mean, come on.

The Confidence Boost You Didn't Know You Needed

It was in that moment that I fully understood the power of makeup and confidence. It wasn't about hiding imperfections or trying to look like someone else. It was about stepping into the best version of myself—feeling good, looking good, and owning my space.

And that's what I want for you too. Whether it's makeup or something else, find what makes you feel really good about yourself. It's not about changing who you are—it's about enhancing what's already there.

Why Makeup Matters (And Why It's More Than Skin Deep)

Let's get one thing straight: makeup isn't superficial. For so many women, it's a form of self-expression, a way to show up for themselves, and a tool for feeling confident. When you feel good about how you look, that confidence radiates into everything you do.

It's like the saying goes: **when you look good, you feel good, and when you feel good, you do good**. That's not just a marketing tagline—it's the truth.

When you invest in yourself, even in small ways like applying makeup, you're sending a message to yourself that you're worth the effort. And that's where confidence begins.

The Ripple Effect: Confidence Creates Action

Here's the secret sauce: confidence isn't just a feeling—it's a catalyst for action. When you feel good about yourself, you're more likely to take on challenges, say yes to opportunities, and show up in bigger, bolder ways.

It's not just about how you look; it's about how you feel. And when you feel really amazing, you start to spread that energy around. You lift others up, offer compliments, and generally make the world a brighter place just by being in it.

In Conclusion: Makeup, Confidence, and the Journey Ahead

So, there it is: makeup isn't just about looking good—it's about feeling good and, ultimately, doing good. It's about boosting your confidence, giving you the power to show up for yourself, and creating a ripple effect that touches everyone around you.

If makeup can help a girl who once thought her teenage heartbreak would haunt her forever stand in front of that same boy 26 years later and feel *amazing*, then it's worth every minute in front of the mirror.

But here's the thing: confidence is just the beginning. In the next chapter, we're diving deeper into what it means to fully embrace your Fit Babe Energy—where strength, discipline, and showing up for yourself every single day becomes your new normal.

Get ready, because confidence is just the foundation. Now, we're about to unleash the full power of your Fit Babe Energy.

Chapter 6

The Power of Showing Up
(For Yourself)

Let's set the record straight: Fit Babe Energy isn't about looking perfect or squeezing into a smaller size. Sure, you might eventually slide into those old jeans, and people might start noticing a certain glow about you—but those are just fringe benefits. The real essence of Fit Babe Energy is much deeper than aesthetics. It's about how you move through life, how you show up for yourself, day in and day out. It's about the unshakable belief that, come what may, you've got this.

Whether it's a mountain of laundry, a brutal work deadline, or the chaos of three kids screaming for attention, Fit Babe Energy gives you the confidence to look at the madness and think, *"Bring it on."* It's sneaking in a few push-ups while waiting for mac and cheese to cook because, let's be honest, that might be the only time you have to move your body that day. It's choosing an apple over chips, not because you're punishing yourself, but because you want to feel good in your own skin. Every small action you take becomes a brick in the foundation of something much bigger.

The Domino Effect of Tiny Wins

We've all been there—caught up in the fantasy of the ultimate fitness goal, that life-changing transformation moment where everything magically falls into place. But here's the truth: those big moments? They don't happen without a hundred tiny wins along the way.

It's the decision to stretch for five minutes before bed when all you really want to do is crash. It's opting for something nourishing when your brain is screaming for junk food. It's waking up just a few minutes earlier, not for anyone else, but because you want to feel good for yourself.

Every one of these choices is like adding a penny to your confidence piggy bank. And trust me, those pennies add up. One day, you'll look back and realize you've built something truly incredible— a deep, unwavering trust in yourself. That's when everything changes. You'll realize you're not just capable of taking on the world—you're unstoppable.

Enter Natelie: The Confidence Queen

Now, I need to tell you about someone who embodies this kind of unshakable confidence and shows up for herself in ways that make you sit up and pay attention. Her name is Natelie, and if you've ever met her, you'll know she's impossible to forget. Natelie's got this larger-than-life personality that stays with you long after she's left the room. You know the type—one of those rare people whose energy makes you smile just thinking about them.

I met Natelie sometime in the last couple of years, though the timeline is fuzzy because her presence is so impactful, it feels like she's always been around. She works for my dear friend Dawn, who runs a hugely successful residential cleaning company. Dawn has been an inspiration to me—so much so that after COVID, I launched my own cleaning business. While Dawn's company handles recurring residential cleaning, mine focuses on commercial work and post-construction cleanups. We've teamed up before, even sharing a booth at a local home show. And that's where the magic of Natelie's confidence came into full bloom.

The Home Show Hustle

Picture this: It's a quiet afternoon at the home show, not many visitors are stopping by. I had brought my oldest son with me, who was nine at the time, and he and Natelie hit it off immediately. They were this hilarious, unstoppable duo. Natelie, always the go-getter, decided that the booth needed more traffic, so she turned to my son and said, *"Let's make people come to us!"*

What happened next was nothing short of genius. Natelie, with all the charisma of a Shirley Temple, grabbed a stack of coupon cards, stepped out into the aisle, and started joyfully announcing,

"WELCOME TO CHILI'S!" The confusion on people's faces was priceless. Their initial *"don't talk to me"* expressions melted into warm laughter, and before we knew it, they were stepping up to the booth, curious about the businesses we were representing.

It wasn't just a gimmick. Natelie was magnetic. She made you feel like you wanted to be part of whatever she was doing. It's that kind of confidence—the *I'm-already-a-star-and-you-don't-even-know-it-yet* confidence—that draws people in. And she didn't stop there.

Owning Her Power

You see, Natelie wasn't always running the show. She started out as one of Dawn's cleaners, but from day one, she told Dawn, *"I'm going to run this company one day and open new locations."* And here's the kicker: she said it with such certainty, such *this-is-already-happening* energy, that it was impossible not to believe her.

Before long, Natelie moved from cleaning to working in the office, and her influence only grew. Her ability to connect with people and her unshakable belief in herself made her an integral part of Dawn's company. It was like watching a masterclass in what happens when you show up for yourself with conviction.

The Natelie Effect

One of the things Natelie told me recently, as we were swapping stories about life and dating, sums her up perfectly. She laughed and said, *"Oh, I just act like everyone I meet is wildly in love with me. So when I talk to them, I kid about how in love with me they are. It throws them off so much, and they always come towards me instead of away. It just works."*

Imagine walking through life with that kind of confidence—that belief that everyone is in love with you. It's not arrogance. It's not self-obsession. It's an unwavering trust in your own worth. Natelie's confidence isn't just something she taps into when things are going well. It's a constant, something she carries with her in every interaction. She's not waiting for permission to be amazing. She just *is*.

Now, think about how transformative that could be. How many of us go through life full of self-doubt, convinced that people don't like us or that we're not worthy of the attention we seek? Natelie's approach is the opposite. She's teaching us that when you *believe* everyone is already in love with you, they start acting like they are. It's not about waiting for someone else to validate your worth; it's about owning it so completely that everyone else catches on.

The Magic of Showing Up—Like Natelie

Here's the thing: Natelie didn't wait for someone to hand her a role in the company or tell her she was good enough to be running things. She showed up with the belief that she was already there. And that's the magic. When you show up for yourself like that, the world responds.

What would happen if you walked through life with the belief that everyone at the table is already in love with you? Can you imagine how differently you'd approach opportunities, relationships, and even your own goals? Instead of constantly second-guessing yourself, you'd show up with the confidence that you belong. Not only that— you'd believe you're *thriving*.

The Domino Effect of Confidence

This is what showing up for yourself looks like in action. It's those small moments, like Natelie stepping into the aisle with a stack of coupons, or me deciding to launch a business when the world felt uncertain. Those moments aren't about grand gestures. They're about a series of tiny decisions—each one building on the next, each one saying, *"I'm worth it."*

Every time you choose to show up for yourself, no matter how small the action, you're reinforcing that you deserve to be here. And that's what Fit Babe Energy is all about. It's not about waiting until you're "ready." It's about stepping into your power, just like Natelie does, and realizing that the only person who needs to believe in you—is you.

The Natelie Lesson: Confidence as a Superpower

When Natelie shows up, she isn't just there for herself—she's influencing everyone around her. She reminds us that confidence isn't about waiting for someone to tell you that you're worthy. It's about walking into a room like you've already won. And here's the kicker—when you believe it, others believe it too. That's the kind of confidence that changes everything.

And if Natelie can do it—so can you.

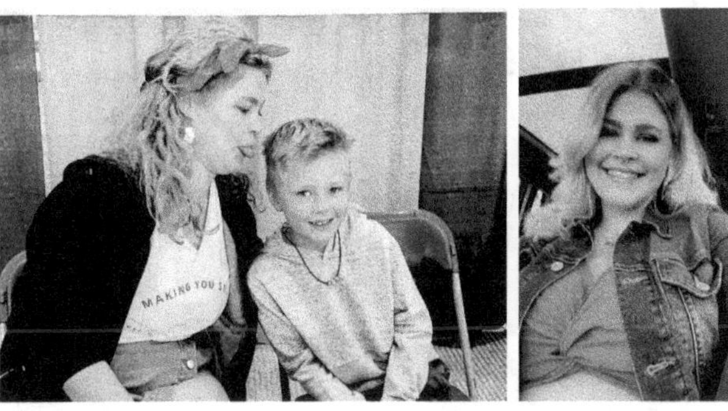

First photo: Natelie being herself with my oldest son at the Home Show

Conclusion: The Power of Showing Up

Here's the real truth: Fit Babe Energy isn't just a workout plan—it's a blueprint for life. It's about building a relationship with yourself that's rooted in trust, love, and respect. It's about showing up in the small moments, over and over again, and watching how those tiny wins add up to something massive.

When you start prioritizing yourself, everything in your life gets better. Your mindset shifts, your relationships improve, and you start living the life you've always dreamed of. Because when you trust yourself, there's nothing you can't achieve.

This is what Fit Babe Energy is all about—embracing it, owning it, and watching how it transforms everything.

Chapter 7

Fueling Your Fit Babe Energy: Ditching Diets and Embracing Real Food

When I hired Jillian, my badass personal trainer with legs that could play sports all on their own, I knew she'd come at me with a nutrition plan. Of course, she did—trainers love that stuff. But I fought it tooth and nail. The last thing I wanted was to be trapped in the soul-sucking cycle of dieting again.

Jillian was adamant, though. "You need to fuel your body properly," she'd say, arms crossed and giving me that look like she was ready to bench press a building. But I wasn't having it. I knew that if I was on a "diet," everything in my being would rebel. I'd been down that road before, and it didn't lead anywhere good.

Still, Jillian wasn't one to take no for an answer. "Fine," she said, "But at least let me share some shopping lists with you." Little did I know that these would be my salvation. She also got me hooked on peanut butter and rice cakes (or on an English muffin). Simple, satisfying, and—most importantly—sustainable. It became my go-to meal, and to this day, it's a staple in my routine. The fewer food decisions I need to make, the easier my life is.

If there's one thing I've learned on this journey, it's that food is not the enemy. We've been conditioned to believe that in order to lose weight or feel good, we have to eat less—fewer calories, fewer carbs, less joy. But food is meant to fuel your body so it can thrive. When you start seeing food as fuel instead of something to fear, your entire relationship with meals changes. And it certainly changed mine.

No More Dieting: Eating for Fit Babe Energy

Let's make this clear: eating for Fit Babe Energy isn't about following some restrictive diet, counting every calorie, or cutting out entire food groups. I'm not here to tell you that keto is the answer or that gluten should be banished forever. Instead, this is about creating a sustainable way of eating that fuels your body, supports your goals, and, most importantly, tastes amazing.

In my journey, I had to unlearn the idea that less food was better. I wasn't going to starve myself anymore or freak out over every bite. Instead, I focused on what my body needed to feel strong and energetic: lean protein, healthy fats, fiber-rich veggies, and just enough carbs to keep my energy up.

The Foundation of Fit Babe Energy: Food That Fuels You

Here's the deal: protein became my best friend. If you're trying to build muscle and lose fat, protein is non-negotiable. It repairs your muscles, helps keep you full, and balances your blood sugar. But protein alone won't cut it—you also need healthy fats to keep your brain sharp and your hormones in check. And let's not forget carbs—yes, carbs! You need them to power through workouts and your everyday hustle. The key is choosing the right kinds of carbs, like whole grains, sweet potatoes, and quinoa, and eating them in the right amounts.

Most importantly? It's about listening to your body. I don't count calories because I trust my body to tell me when it's full. I focus on intuitive eating—tuning in to my hunger cues and stopping when I'm satisfied, not stuffed.

A Simple Grocery List for Fit Babe Energy

Jillian's shopping lists were the first step to simplifying my life. Eating for Fit Babe Energy doesn't require fancy ingredients or complex recipes. You don't need to be a gourmet chef. All of what you need can be found at your local grocery store, and the best part? You can mix and match meals depending on what's on your schedule or what you're craving that day.

Here's a basic grocery list that's simple and effective:

Proteins:

- Chicken breast (4-5 lbs)

- Ground turkey (2-3 lbs)

- Salmon fillets (4-6)

- White fish (e.g., tilapia or cod)

- Eggs (2 dozen)

- Greek yogurt (plain, nonfat) – 2 large tubs

- Cottage cheese (low-fat) – 2 tubs

- Tofu (optional)

- Protein powder (including unflavored Protein Powder to sneak into recipes)

Carbs:

- Rice Cakes (plain or white cheddar)

- Whole grain bread or English muffins (multigrain)

- Brown rice (1-2 bags)

- Quinoa (1-2 bags)

- Sweet potatoes (6-8)

- Oats (1 large tub)

Veggies & Fruits:

- Leafy greens (spinach, kale)
- Broccoli (3-4 heads)
- Bell peppers (3-4)
- Zucchini (3-4)
- Asparagus (2-3 bunches)
- Apples (7-10)
- Berries (frozen or fresh)

Healthy Fats:

- Natural Peanut butter (2 jars)
- Almonds, walnuts (small bag for snacks)
- Avocado (4-6)
- Olive oil (for cooking)

Miscellaneous:

- Lemon, garlic, spices (cumin, paprika, chili powder, etc.)
- Low-sodium soy sauce
- Hot sauce or salsa
- Unsweetened almond milk

Peanut Butter and English Muffins: The Unsung Hero

Let me tell you, there's a lot of buzz around "superfoods" these days—chia seeds, kale smoothies, you name it. But for me? My secret weapon isn't some obscure grain grown in the mountains of Tibet. It's peanut butter and an English muffin. Groundbreaking, right? Well, it kind of is.

My mom always jokes, "You must be doing something right if you're losing weight and getting toned while eating peanut butter and English muffins all the time!" And she's got a point. Jillian, my powerhouse trainer, was the one who first suggested it. She looked me dead in the eye and said, "Peanut butter and rice cakes or an English muffin—simple, filling, and perfect for lifting." No quinoa, no kale—just straight-up, no-nonsense fuel. Don't get me wrong, I do love some quinoa and kale, but that takes way more effort than this simple hack!

And guess what? It works. This combo is the perfect trifecta: protein to rebuild those muscles, healthy fats to keep you satisfied, and carbs to give you the energy to lift heavier without crashing by 3 p.m. It's like the holy grail of snacks disguised as comfort food.

The best part? There's no mental Olympics over "What should I eat today?" It's right there—simple, delicious, and zero stress. Forget spending hours meal-prepping like you're on *Top Chef.*

Peanut butter and an English muffin get the job done without the drama. Plus, it keeps me full long enough to survive a workout and three kids.

So while some people are out there choking down celery juice, I'm over here enjoying my peanut butter English muffin, feeling like I've cracked the secret to life. Sure, it may not win any "clean eating" awards, but hey, if it's keeping me toned and sane, I'll take it.

Two-Week Meal Plan for Fit Babe Energy

This meal plan isn't a diet. It's a guide to fueling your body in a way that helps you lose weight, build muscle, and feel amazing—all without deprivation. It's balanced, high in protein, and full of nutrient-dense foods that keep you satisfied and energized.

Here's how you can structure your meals over two weeks, with peanut butter on English muffins making regular appearances, of course:

Week 1

Day 1

- **Breakfast**: Scrambled eggs with spinach and avocado
- **Snack**: Greek yogurt with berries
- **Lunch**: Grilled chicken salad with mixed greens, cucumber, and olive oil dressing
- **Snack**: Apple with peanut butter

- **Dinner**: Baked salmon with roasted sweet potatoes and asparagus

Day 2

- **Breakfast**: Peanut butter on a whole grain English muffin, topped with banana slices
- **Snack**: Cottage cheese with sliced cucumbers
- **Lunch**: Turkey meatballs with quinoa and broccoli
- **Snack**: Handful of almonds
- **Dinner**: Grilled tilapia with brown rice and sautéed zucchini

Day 3

- **Breakfast**: Protein smoothie with almond milk, protein powder, spinach, and a handful of berries
- **Snack**: Hard-boiled eggs
- **Lunch**: Grilled chicken with quinoa and roasted veggies
- **Snack**: Carrot sticks with hummus
- **Dinner**: Ground turkey stir-fry with bell peppers and broccoli

Day 4

- **Breakfast**: Oatmeal topped with almonds and a dollop of peanut butter
- **Snack**: Cottage cheese with a handful of berries

- **Lunch**: Tuna salad with mixed greens, olive oil, and vinegar dressing
- **Snack**: Cucumber slices and avocado
- **Dinner**: Baked chicken breast with sweet potato fries and sautéed green beans

Day 5

- **Breakfast**: Peanut butter on an English muffin with sliced strawberries
- **Snack**: Greek yogurt with chia seeds
- **Lunch**: Grilled turkey burger (no bun) with a side of salad
- **Snack**: Apple slices with almond butter
- **Dinner**: Baked cod with quinoa and steamed broccoli

Day 6

- **Breakfast**: Veggie omelet with mushrooms, spinach, and bell peppers
- **Snack**: Cottage cheese with a few walnuts
- **Lunch**: Leftover turkey stir-fry with brown rice
- **Snack**: Carrot sticks with peanut butter
- **Dinner**: Grilled salmon with roasted Brussels sprouts

Day 7

- **Breakfast**: Peanut butter on an English muffin with a side of Greek yogurt
- **Snack**: Protein smoothie with almond milk, spinach, and berries
- **Lunch**: Grilled chicken salad with avocado and olive oil dressing
- **Snack**: Apple with peanut butter
- **Dinner**: Ground turkey chili with diced tomatoes, beans, and bell peppers

Week 2 (Examples)

Day 8

- **Breakfast**: Scrambled eggs with avocado and salsa
- **Snack**: Greek yogurt with berries
- **Lunch**: Grilled tilapia with quinoa and steamed broccoli
- **Snack**: Carrot sticks with hummus
- **Dinner**: Baked chicken breast with roasted sweet potatoes and asparagus

Day 9

- **Breakfast**: Peanut butter on a whole grain English muffin, topped with banana slices
- **Snack**: Cottage cheese with sliced cucumbers
- **Lunch**: Ground turkey stir-fry with bell peppers and spinach
- **Snack**: Hard-boiled eggs
- **Dinner**: Baked salmon with a side of mixed greens salad

Day 10

- **Breakfast**: Protein smoothie with almond milk, protein powder, spinach, and berries
- **Snack**: Apple with peanut butter
- **Lunch**: Chicken breast with brown rice and steamed zucchini
- **Snack**: Greek yogurt with chia seeds
- **Dinner**: Grilled cod with roasted Brussels sprouts

Day 11

- **Breakfast**: Oatmeal topped with almonds and a dollop of peanut butter
- **Snack**: Cottage cheese with berries
- **Lunch**: Leftover turkey chili with salad greens
- **Snack**: Cucumber slices with hummus
- **Dinner**: Grilled chicken with quinoa and roasted veggies

Day 12

- **Breakfast**: Peanut butter on an English muffin with strawberries
- **Snack**: Protein smoothie with almond milk, spinach, and berries
- **Lunch**: Grilled turkey burger (no bun) with a side salad
- **Snack**: Handful of almonds
- **Dinner**: Baked cod with sweet potato fries and sautéed green beans

Day 13

- **Breakfast**: Veggie omelet with mushrooms, spinach, and bell peppers
- **Snack**: Hard-boiled eggs
- **Lunch**: Grilled chicken salad with avocado and olive oil dressing
- **Snack**: Greek yogurt with a handful of berries
- **Dinner**: Ground turkey stir-fry with bell peppers and quinoa

Day 14

- **Breakfast**: Peanut butter on an English muffin with Greek yogurt on the side
- **Snack**: Cottage cheese with cucumber slices

- **Lunch**: Grilled salmon with brown rice and steamed broccoli

- **Snack**: Apple with peanut butter

- **Dinner**: Baked chicken breast with roasted Brussels sprouts and sweet potatoes

Why I Don't Count Calories (And You Don't Have To Either)

For years, I was convinced that the only way to lose weight was by counting every single calorie. It felt like I was at war with myself—constantly thinking about food, constantly worrying about going over my calorie "limit." It was exhausting, unsustainable, and—most importantly—it wasn't working.

That's when I made the decision to let go of calorie counting altogether. Instead, I focused on eating intuitively. I started tuning in to my body's hunger cues and learning how to trust myself around food. I ate when I was hungry, stopped when I was full, and focused on nutrient-dense meals that made me feel strong and energized.

The result? I lost weight, built muscle, and—perhaps most importantly—I stopped stressing about food. The key is balance, not restriction. When you fuel your body with the right foods, it knows exactly what to do with them.

In Conclusion: Fueling for Fit Babe Energy

Eating for Fit Babe Energy isn't about deprivation—it's about fueling your body so it can thrive. It's about enjoying your meals, nourishing your muscles, and feeling strong, energized, and unstoppable throughout the day.

The meal plan and grocery list I've shared here are just a starting point. They're designed to give you the tools you need to fuel your body without stress, without deprivation, and without the endless cycle of dieting. Remember, this journey isn't about perfection. It's about making small, consistent choices that help you feel your best.

Now that we've covered how to fuel your body, it's time to dive deeper into how to train for success. In the next chapter, we'll explore the workouts that build strength, boost confidence, and help you unleash your full Fit Babe Energy.

Chapter 8

Lessons from Perimenopause – The Hormone Hustle (and Why Sugar and Alcohol are Not Your Friends)

Let's talk about something no one ever brings up in their 20s: hormones. Back then, I was sure I was invincible. Eating pizza at midnight, staying up late, bouncing back from anything like I was made of rubber. Fast forward a couple of decades, and I found myself standing on the tracks of a freight train called perimenopause—without a manual or even a heads-up.

The Hormone Freight Train

One day, I was in my 40s, juggling three boys, running businesses, and working hard to keep my fitness journey on track. I thought I had it all figured out: eat clean, work out, practice self-care. But then, it was like someone flipped a switch. My body stopped responding the way it used to. The weight wouldn't budge despite my best efforts. It was like my body had turned into some kind of energy-sucking parasite.

Cue the mood swings, crying fits, and sleepless nights. I'd wake up at 3 a.m., wide awake, grappling with an existential dread that came out of nowhere. One minute, I'd be laughing, and the next,

I'd snap at someone for asking what's for breakfast. Yep, the good ol' perimenopausal emotional rollercoaster. It felt like my body was conspiring against me.

But instead of getting angry, I decided to do something different: I started listening to my body. And that's when everything began to change.

The Wake-Up Call: Learning to Listen (Not Fight)

Perimenopause taught me one of life's most valuable lessons: your body is always talking to you. It's like a constant stream of signals, telling you what it needs, what's off, and where it needs extra care. The problem? Most of us spend our lives ignoring those signals or silencing them with diet fads, endless cups of coffee, and sheer willpower. I was guilty of it for years.

My go-to solution for everything had always been "do more." More workouts, stricter diets, more discipline. But guess what? Perimenopause doesn't care about your hustle. The harder I pushed, the more my body pushed back. It wasn't until I stopped trying to control everything that things finally started to click.

I let go of counting calories and ditched the rigid diets. Instead, I started listening—really listening. When I was hungry, I ate. When I was tired, I rested. When I craved something sweet, I didn't beat myself up (okay, more on sugar in a minute). I stopped treating my body like an enemy and started working with it.

Sugar and Alcohol: The Frenemies You Don't Need

Now, let's talk about sugar and alcohol. I know, I know—don't kill the messenger—but the truth is, sugar is your enemy. Seriously, it's like feeding poison to your body. It fuels disease, wreaks havoc on your hormones, and messes with your hunger cues, making you crave more and more. And alcohol? Well, it's literally a toxin. I'm not saying you have to quit cold turkey, but you need to be aware of the effects they have on your body.

Think of sugar and alcohol as those frenemies who act sweet to your face but stab you in the back. They seem innocent enough in moderation, but when consumed regularly, they disrupt your hormones and slow down your metabolism. Trust me—I've been there. I used to love a glass of Riesling with dinner or a gin and tonic on the weekends, but I had to set some boundaries.

I cut out blatant sugar—no more sugar in my coffee, no more dessert after dinner—and you know what? I didn't miss it. When you're off sugar, your body stops craving it. You feel so much better. Same goes for alcohol. I didn't quit drinking entirely, but I became a lot more intentional about when I indulged. The result? My hormones balanced out, my metabolism woke up, and my body started functioning the way it was supposed to.

Am I telling you never to enjoy a drink again? Absolutely not. But if you limit sugar and alcohol, your hormones stabilize, your metabolism gets a break, and your body gets the fuel it needs to function at its best.

The Metabolism Myth: Eat More, Weigh Less

Back in my 20s, I could eat a pizza at midnight and still wake up with a flat stomach. Once I hit 39, though, my metabolism slowed to a crawl. No matter how many carbs I cut or how much I worked out, nothing budged. My body was hoarding fat like it was preparing for the apocalypse.

Here's the kicker: my body wasn't the problem. My mindset was. I was treating my 40+ body like it was still 20, punishing it with restrictions and over-exercising. But guess what? You can't bully your body into submission, especially not during perimenopause. The more I deprived myself, the more my body resisted.

Then, I had an epiphany: maybe my body needed more fuel, not less. I started eating more—more protein, more healthy fats, and yes, even carbs. I began to nourish my body instead of depriving it, and guess what happened? My metabolism fired up like a rocket.

Learning to Eat Like a Grown-Up

In my 20s, I could survive on snacks and coffee and still feel invincible. But those days are long gone. If you want to thrive during perimenopause, you have to start eating like an adult. No more junk food binges, no more living off caffeine.

For me, protein became my new best friend. Chicken, fish, eggs, and Greek yogurt became staples in my diet. Protein helps stabilize your blood sugar, supports muscle repair, and keeps you full longer. I also embraced healthy fats—avocados, olive oil, nuts. These fats aren't the villains they've been made out to be. They're essential for hormone balance and brain health.

And carbs? They're not the enemy either. Cutting out carbs won't solve your problems. Your body needs them for energy. The key is choosing the right kinds of carbs—whole grains, quinoa, sweet potatoes—that give you sustained energy without causing blood sugar spikes.

The Power of Hormone-Friendly Foods

Let's talk about the foods that really matter—the ones that keep your hormones in check. Perimenopause is like a hormonal whirlwind, and what you eat can either help or hinder the process.

Here are some hormone-friendly superheroes:

- **Salmon**: Rich in omega-3s, great for reducing inflammation and supporting brain health.

- **Leafy greens**: Spinach, kale, and other dark greens are packed with nutrients that support hormone balance and liver function.

- **Flaxseeds**: These tiny seeds are hormone-balancing powerhouses, full of lignans that help regulate estrogen.

- **Berries**: Loaded with antioxidants that reduce oxidative stress and help your hormones stay balanced.

The Moment I Stopped Counting Calories

I'd been a calorie-counting maniac for years, obsessing over every bite. But after a while, it became clear that it wasn't helping anymore. It was exhausting—mentally, physically, emotionally. I'd spend entire days calculating numbers in my head, and for what? Misery?

So, I stopped. I threw the calorie counter out the window and decided to start trusting my body. I ate when I was hungry, stopped when I was full, and focused on the quality of my food, not the quantity. And guess what? It worked. Without the constant stress of counting every bite, my body finally found its rhythm. I lost weight, my metabolism picked up, and I felt better than ever.

How Perimenopause Made Me Stronger

Perimenopause isn't the enemy. In fact, it's an opportunity to learn more about your body than ever before. Sure, it comes with challenges (hello, mood swings), but it also comes with the chance to build a stronger relationship with yourself.

This phase of life taught me that my body needs different things now. It's not about punishment or restriction anymore. It's about working with my body, respecting its signals, and thriving through it all. The more I embraced that mindset, the stronger I became.

Guess What?: My Metabolism Is Stronger Than Ever

After years of frustration, I cracked the code. My metabolism isn't broken—it's just evolved. By focusing on nourishment rather than deprivation, and by cutting out sugar and limiting alcohol, I gave my body what it needed to thrive. And now? My metabolism is stronger than ever.

Embracing the Hormone Hustle: The Final Word

Perimenopause taught me that my body is constantly evolving, and it's not something to fear. It's a new chapter where you learn to nourish, respect, and trust yourself more than ever before. The hormone hustle isn't about fighting your body—it's about working with it, fueling it right, and thriving through every change.

Sugar and alcohol? They're not your friends. They might seem harmless, but cutting them back—or cutting them out—can be one of the best gifts you can give yourself. Your hormones, metabolism, and future self will thank you.

Here's to listening to your body, embracing the hormone hustle, and discovering that you're stronger, healthier, and more powerful than you ever imagined.

Now, let's dive deeper, because Fit Babe Energy is just getting started, and so are you.

Chapter 9

The 10 Commandments of Happiness

I remember it like it was yesterday. There I was, standing in the middle of my kitchen, staring blankly at the fridge. The kids were screaming, my phone was buzzing, and there was a half-written email waiting for me—but all I could think was, *What am I even doing?* I felt like I was spinning in circles, pulled in a million different directions with no sense of where I was actually headed. Sure, I was surviving, but thriving? Not even close.

Then it hit me like a ton of bricks: I had no idea what I really wanted out of life. I was just floating along, reacting to whatever came my way. I needed to figure out what I truly wanted, not just what everyone else expected from me.

This is where Fit Babe Energy truly kicks in. It's not just about lifting weights or building muscle—it's about getting clear on your goals, your desires, and the things that set your soul on fire. It's about creating a roadmap for your life, making sure that every choice you make aligns with that vision.

So, I did something radical: I took a few days for myself. I shut out the noise, ignored my texts, and spent some serious time thinking about what I wanted *for me*. And that's when the 10 Commandments of Happiness came to life. These weren't just goals—they were guiding principles, the pillars that would shape my path forward.

Distractions Are Everywhere—But You Can't Go Anywhere Without a Map

Here's the hard truth: distractions are *everywhere*. Social media, work, family obligations, Netflix—everything is designed to pull you in a million directions. And if you don't know what you want, it's easy to get sucked into it all. You start saying "yes" to things that don't really matter, and before you know it, your days are filled with stuff that's completely out of alignment with who you are.

I was there. I was saying "yes" to everything, thinking I had to be everything to everyone. But here's what I realized: without a clear sense of what I wanted, I was never going to get where I wanted to go. I needed a roadmap.

It's like trying to take a road trip without a GPS. Sure, you'll end up *somewhere*, but it's probably not where you wanted to be. You need a destination. So, I started writing down my goals—not the fluffy, vague kind like "be happy" or "get fit," but real, specific, actionable goals that got me out of bed in the morning.

The 10 Commandments of Happiness

Once I started writing, it became clear that certain areas of my life needed serious attention. I couldn't just focus on one thing and expect the rest to magically fall into place. Every part of my life— physical health, emotional well-being, relationships, finances, passions—needed to be in balance if I wanted to live with true Fit Babe Energy.

That's when I created the *10 Commandments of Happiness*. These aren't just guidelines for me—they're a roadmap for my life, and more than that, I hope they can be a guide for you too. This book? It's not about telling you what I want or how I've figured things out. It's about giving you the tools to fill out your own version of what lights *you* up, what *you* really want.

I've walked this path, stumbled more times than I can count, and through it all, I've learned a lot. But I'm not here to tell you that my way is the only way. Instead, I'm offering what I've discovered so you can learn how to fill out those sections in your life that might feel neglected or incomplete. This book? It's for you. You're the reason I'm sharing all of this—not because I've got it all together, but because I've been where you are, and I want to help you find your way too.

These *10 Commandments of Happiness* became my guiding principles, helping me stay focused on what really matters. I hope they give you the same sense of clarity and direction as you move through your own journey of discovering what lights you up and what truly makes you happy. So, let's break them down.

1. Physical/Fitness: What Do I Want for My Body?

This one's obvious, right? It's called *Fit Babe Energy* for a reason! But for me, it wasn't just about hitting the gym or dropping a few pounds—it was about truly understanding what I wanted my body to *feel* like. I wasn't chasing some unattainable, airbrushed body standard. Instead, I wanted to feel strong, capable, and genuinely confident in my own skin.

But here's the kicker: I got specific. I set real, tangible goals. I decided I wanted to develop round glutes within two years (yes, the booty is a top priority) and get myself a six-pack of abs. Totally doable. I wasn't playing around with vague wishes anymore—I had a clear vision.

I planned out my workouts, my nutrition, and made sure to prioritize rest and recovery, which is just as crucial as the reps. I stopped obsessing over the number on the scale and started focusing on how my body felt after a workout, how energized I was, and how strong I was becoming.

And that shift? It changed everything. I wasn't at war with my body anymore—I was working with it, fueling it, and trusting it to get me where I wanted to go. Now, every squat, every lunge, and every bite of food has a purpose—and it feels damn good.

2. Spiritual: How Do I Connect With Something Greater Than Myself?

This one wasn't as tricky for me as it might be for some. I'm a Christian, and my faith in God and Jesus has always been an important part of my life. But I'll admit, in the chaos of raising kids, building businesses, and staying on top of everything else, I hadn't given my spiritual well-being the time and attention it needed.

I realized that if I wanted to live with true Fit Babe Energy, I had to reconnect with my faith. It wasn't about some "woo woo" practice or chasing after spiritual trends. For me, it meant carving out intentional time for prayer and grounding myself in God's truth. Sometimes it was as simple as stepping outside, taking a deep breath, and remembering that I'm part of a bigger plan—one that's far beyond my to-do list or the daily grind. In those moments, I found peace and a renewed sense of purpose.

3. Romantic Relationship: What Do I Want From My Partner?

For the first time, I took a step back and really examined my needs in a romantic relationship—something I'd never done intentionally before. What did I, Chrissy, want? Did I even want to get married again? I decided it was time to dig deep and ask myself the tough questions.

For years, I had been so focused on taking care of everyone else that I never stopped to think about what I needed from a relationship. I had just been coasting along, hoping things would work out on their own. But hope isn't a strategy. I realized that if I wanted to be happy, I needed to define what that looked like for me.

So, I got real. I asked myself, "What kind of partnership do I want? How do I want to feel with my partner?" The answer was clear: I wanted a relationship where I felt truly seen, heard, valued, and supported. Someone who was not just physically present, but emotionally in it together where we lifted each other up and poured life and love into each other while we also took the time to make sure our own cup was full.

But here's the kicker—I also decided, for the first time, to have expectations of people, especially in a romantic relationship. This was something I had always been terrified of before. I had lived with the belief that if you don't have expectations of others, you won't get hurt. No expectations, no disappointment, right? But here's the truth: living that way also keeps you from experiencing the depth of life. It keeps you from having meaningful connections, from growing, and from knowing who's truly right for you.

By finally having expectations—both of myself and of the people around me—I started to see things more clearly. I could then decide what relationships would stay in my life and what had to go. When you start living intentionally and set standards for how you want to be treated, you gain the power to choose who belongs in your story.

This shift wasn't just about romance, either. It applied to every relationship in my life. I stopped settling for what you don't want in friendships, in work, and in love. And that's when everything started to shift—when I embraced the idea that it's important to have expectations, and it's even more than okay to say goodbye to anything that doesn't meet them.

Before we move on, I want to say that a major issue I've had in my life is not speaking up or having a conversation about wants, needs and expectations. From a first date to a long term relationship. I didn't want to be uncomfortable and I didn't want to make my partner uncomfortable, but behavior like this will surely cause resentment in your life and relationships. It is your responsibility to communicate firmly, but without blame your entire list of your own 10 commandments to your partner and invite them to not only write them for themselves but then bring them to you once they do. It will be one of the most rewarding experiences of your relationship!

4. Financial: What Does Financial Freedom Look Like to Me?

Let me be real with you—sitting down and doing the financial stuff scared me. It always seemed like something I could put off or let someone else handle. But here's the truth: there wasn't anyone else coming to save me. It was just me, and that meant everything I needed had to come from what I built, from what I created. That's an empowering realization, but it also comes with a dose of fear.

For too long, I avoided these conversations, even when I was married or in long-term relationships. We'd dance around money like it was some taboo subject, never really sitting down and hashing out the details. But I've learned that if you want real freedom—real control over your life—you have to face it head-on. No more skirting the issue, no more hoping it would work itself out. Financial clarity is power.

So, I sat down, took a deep breath, and mapped it out. What does financial freedom look like for *me*? How much do I actually need to live comfortably? What are my long-term goals? It wasn't just about making more money—it was about building a life where I didn't have to constantly worry about it. I realized that financial freedom for me meant having the security to take care of my family, travel, and pursue my passions without feeling the weight of financial stress hanging over my head.

And listen, I'm single right now, but that doesn't mean I'm not thinking ahead. If the day comes when I decide to marry again or join paths with someone, you can bet those financial goals and plans will be on the table. No more living separately, financially speaking. We'll talk about money, openly and honestly, from the start. Because I've learned that avoiding those conversations doesn't protect you—it only sets you up for problems down the line. Having those tough talks is part of owning your life, your future, and your freedom.

So, I stopped seeing money as this elusive goal and started seeing it as a tool. A tool that can create the life I want if I'm intentional about it. Whether that's building a business, setting up a debt layoff plan, or making smart spending decisions, I know now that my financial future is in my hands—and that's both terrifying and exhilarating.

5. Family: What Do I Want for My Kids?

This one hit me deep. My kids are my world, no question about that, but I realized I didn't want every day with them to feel like *Groundhog Day*—just going through the motions. I needed to be more intentional about the kind of parent I wanted to be, not just someone enforcing rules and routines. I didn't want to run a household that felt like an authoritarian regime, where I laid down the law and expected everyone to fall in line. That's not the vibe I'm going for.

What I want is a family where we can all flourish in our own unique ways, where my boys feel like they have a voice and can express who they are. I don't want to push my beliefs or expectations on them about how they should live their lives. Instead, I want us to talk—really talk—about what we each want, what's important to us, and how we can support each other's individual gifts. My role as their mom isn't to mold them into mini versions of myself; it's to guide them, give them the tools they need to navigate life, and encourage them to be the best version of *themselves*.

That doesn't mean there are no boundaries or that the house is chaos—far from it. I believe in setting healthy boundaries because I want them to understand the importance of discipline and respect. But I also want them to learn independence. I want them to feel empowered to make their own decisions, to try things out, make mistakes, and grow from those experiences.

And here's the kicker—I realized that if I want my kids to grow up into healthy, well-rounded individuals, I have to model what that looks like. I can't run myself ragged, sacrificing my own well-being in the name of being a "good mom," and expect them to somehow prioritize their own self-care. They need to see me taking care of myself—mentally, emotionally, and physically—so they understand that it's not selfish to make yourself a priority.

I want them to see that living intentionally isn't just about crossing things off a to-do list or making it through the day. It's about creating a life that feels fulfilling, where you're aligned with your values and your passions. And I want that for them just as much as I want it for myself. We're a team, and part of being a team means talking things out, supporting each other, and making sure that everyone—myself included—gets the space and encouragement to thrive.

6. Passion: What Lights Me Up?

This one took me a long time to figure out. As an entrepreneur, my passion has always been business. I'm driven, I love the hustle, and building something from the ground up absolutely lights a fire in me. But at some point, I realized I had gotten so wrapped up in the grind, in making things work and bringing in income, that I had lost touch with the things that brought me joy purely for the sake of joy.

I had to sit down and really ask myself: *What lights me up?* What gets me excited when there's no paycheck involved? And you know what ended up on the list? Writing.

Yeah, writing! Who knew, right? I mean, here we are, with me pouring my heart into this book, and it feels like I'm living out one of my dreams. Writing has always been a quiet passion for me, something that I've done in the background—journaling, drafting ideas, putting words to paper just to clear my head. But when I gave myself the space to acknowledge it, to say, "Hey, this brings me joy," it opened up a whole new world. And now, here I am, not just thinking about it or dreaming about it—but doing it. Writing this book has been a full-circle moment for me, like I'm finally stepping into something I've loved all along but never gave myself permission to pursue fully.

And it's not just writing. It's working out, too—that's another passion that keeps me grounded, keeps me feeling strong and alive.

It's something I do not just for the physical benefits, but because it clears my mind, boosts my mood, and makes me feel capable of handling whatever life throws at me. Then there's my passion for helping other women find their confidence. That's what gets me out of bed in the morning, the reason behind so much of what I do. Watching women step into their power, realize their worth, and transform their lives? That's the ultimate reward.

These things—writing, fitness, supporting other women—they're not just tasks on a checklist. They're the things that light me up, that make me feel fully alive. And I had to make space for them in my life, not just because they bring me joy, but because they're part of who I am.

So, I had to ask myself: How do I prioritize these passions, even when they don't necessarily bring in income or fit neatly into my day-to-day grind? The answer was simple but profound: I had to give myself permission to pursue them, no strings attached. I had to remind myself that it's okay to do something just because it makes you happy, that not everything has to have a financial or practical outcome attached to it.

And now? Now, I'm living out my dreams. I'm writing, I'm building, I'm creating—and most importantly, I'm letting myself enjoy the ride. I'm living proof that when you lean into your passions, even the ones that seem like they don't "fit" into your life, magic happens. And that's what keeps me going every day.

7. Business: What Are My Business Goals?

As an entrepreneur with multiple businesses, I had been in constant go-mode, always building, always pushing. But when I finally sat down to reflect, I realized I hadn't truly defined what I *really* wanted out of each business. What was the long-term vision? Where was I steering the ship? And most importantly, did I want to add new ventures or avenues to explore?

This section became one of my favorites to dive into because it allowed me to dream bigger and get incredibly specific about businesses I was connected to. I got clear on each business—what was its purpose? Where was it heading? Did I want to expand any part of it? Should we add new offerings or dive into fresh markets?

And then, the million-dollar question: Was I ready to take on new business ventures altogether? You bet I was. I love the hustle, and the thrill of creating something new was calling my name. But I didn't want to dive in blindly. I wanted each decision to be intentional, aligned with my bigger vision of helping other women step into their power, just like I had.

Once I mapped it all out, I felt a renewed sense of purpose. Each business had a clear direction, and everything I worked on started aligning with my goals. Expansion became not just a possibility but a strategic plan. This wasn't just about running a successful business anymore—it was about making a lasting impact and creating space for growth and new opportunities.

8. Home: What Kind of Home Life Do I Want to Create?

Home is where we recharge and find peace—or at least it should be. For a while, my home felt like pure chaos, and I knew I had to make changes. I wanted a space where both the kids and I could feel calm, safe, and secure. So, I got intentional about routines and structure.

I created a daily schedule that gave us all a sense of stability—mornings with calm moments, an after-school routine that was organized but flexible, and evenings focused on connection. It's not about perfection but reducing chaos where I can and embracing flexibility where it counts.

More importantly, I wanted my kids to feel safe—emotionally and physically. We started having regular family talks to build trust and openness. I also set consistent boundaries, like bedtimes and screen limits, while allowing room for individuality and growth. It's about creating a space where we all feel supported and can thrive together, not just survive the day-to-day grind.

9. Fears: What Fears Are Holding Me Back?

Addressing my fears was a non-negotiable part of this process. Every step of the way, old doubts crept in—before, during, and after writing out what I wanted from life. The biggest fear? That I wasn't enough. I worried I wasn't capable of achieving the life I was dreaming about, that I'd fall short, or worse, fail entirely.

But here's the thing: facing those fears head-on was the only way to move forward. I had to acknowledge the fear of failure, the fear of judgment, and the fear of not living up to my own expectations. Instead of letting those fears paralyze me, I used them as fuel. Each time I felt fear rise up, I reminded myself that I had a choice: to stay stuck or push through.

The truth is, fear doesn't disappear—you just get better at working with it. And each time I confronted those fears, I got stronger, more confident, and more sure of the life I was creating. Fear became a stepping stone, not a roadblock.

10. Lessons: What Has This Process Taught Me?

Writing out exactly what I wanted from life has been one of the most transformative experiences. The biggest lesson? You are the author of your own life. It's easy to drift along, letting life happen to you, but this process taught me that I have the power to actively shape my story. Every choice, every action, every goal is mine to define.

Yes, life will throw curveballs, and things won't always go as planned, but that's part of the journey. What I've learned is that clarity brings empowerment. When you get clear about what you want, you stop reacting to life and start living with intention. This process reminded me that I'm capable of building the life I envision—and the only limits are the ones I set for myself.

In Conclusion: Get Clear on What You Want and Protect Your Fit Babe Energy

The 10 Commandments of Happiness became my personal roadmap, guiding me through every decision, every moment of doubt, and every new opportunity. Once I got clear on what I really wanted, everything else started to fall into place. It wasn't magic—it was intentional living. I cut out distractions, set firm boundaries, and focused on the things that truly mattered to me. And you know what? It worked.

That's what Fit Babe Energy is all about. It's not just about hitting the gym hard or sticking to a perfect diet—it's about aligning your entire life with your values, passions, and purpose. It's about protecting your energy like the precious resource it is and using it to create a life that fires you up every day.

So here's my challenge to you: Take some time for yourself. Get quiet. Block out the noise, the expectations, the obligations, and really ask yourself: What do you want? Write it down. Be specific. Because once you have that clarity, you can start living a life that is fully, unapologetically yours.

And here's the best part: When you start living with that kind of intention, there's no stopping you. You'll be unstoppable—not because life will suddenly get easy, but because you'll know exactly where you're going and what you're willing to fight for. That's Fit Babe Energy. So go out there and claim it. The life you want is waiting.

Chapter 10

Protecting Your Fit Babe Energy – How to Stop Letting Outside Influences Drain You Dry

Here's a little secret nobody tells you when you decide to level up your life: the world is full of energy vampires. They're everywhere, just waiting to suck the life out of you the minute you let your guard down. And it's not just people—it's your phone, social media, that endless group chat, the news, all of it. It's a slow drip of your energy being siphoned off, and if you're not careful, you'll find yourself drained, exhausted, and wondering why you feel like you've been run over before finishing your first cup of coffee.

But here's the thing about Fit Babe Energy: it's not just about how much you can squat or how flawless you look in your favorite leggings. It's about knowing when to protect your vibe, when to throw up boundaries like a steel wall, and when to hang up that "Do Not Disturb" sign on your life. Because if you don't protect your energy, something—or someone—else will.

Buckle up, babe. This chapter is all about reclaiming your energy, protecting your vibe, and keeping that Fit Babe Energy topped up—without sacrificing your sanity.

Start a Diary, But Not the 'Dear Diary' Kind

No, I'm not talking about your teenage journal with a glittery cover. I'm talking about a Fit Babe Energy Diary—a log that tracks your workouts, emotions, and, most importantly, your energy. It's become my personal sanity-saver, where I put everything from my fitness journey to how I'm feeling mentally.

Here's what it looks like:

- **Day of the Week**: Mondays hit different than Fridays, don't they?

- **Date**: For tracking trends and patterns.

- **Legs/Push/Pull**: What body part or movement pattern I'm working on that day.

- **Weight**: No, not my body weight—we're talking about the weights I'm lifting, and yes, they're getting heavier.

- **Feeling**: This is the magic ingredient. Am I feeling like a beast or like I want to curl up in a ball and cry? It's all here.

- **Cycle Day**: I track my cycle with an app because hormones can explain so much, like why I'm ready to conquer the world on some days and on others, I'm crying over avocados being out of stock.

- **Workout**: The nitty-gritty—sets, reps, weights.

Here's an example of one of my actual logs:

Sunday 7/2 - Pull

144

Cycle Day 17

Feeling: Sadness. Anger. But it pushes me to keep going. Called Candace about makeup stuff, cried for no reason. THIS KIND OF SHIT KEEPS HAPPENING, AND I WILL IT, PRAY FOR IT TO STOP.

Stair Stepper: 5 min

Hammer Curl: 15 lb - 1x15, 12 (failure), 12, 9 (failure)

Tricep Pull-down: 50 lb - 1x15, 15, 14, 12

Wide Grip Lat Pull-down: 65 lb - 1x15 / 85 lb - 1x12, 11, 10

Underhand Narrow Grip: 85 lb - 1x15, 15, 14, 12 (forearm failure)

Keeping this log was a game-changer for me. It stopped being about beating myself up for having "off days" and instead, I started spotting trends. Oh, it's Day 22 of my cycle? No wonder I feel like sobbing through leg day. By understanding my body and my patterns, I stopped blaming myself and started working *with* my energy, not against it.

Lifting Weights and Crying – Totally Normal

Here's a fun fact they don't mention in fitness magazines: Lifting heavy might make you cry. Not from muscle pain, but from *life* pain. You know, the "why is everything falling apart" kind of cry.

I remember the first time it happened. I was deep into a set of skull crushers when, out of nowhere, the tears came. And not a dainty tear, but full-on sobbing. It was like my emotions got mixed into the workout and suddenly, everything came pouring out. I Googled it later and found out that crying during or after lifting is actually normal. Lifting heavy activates your nervous system and sometimes, the emotional floodgates just open.

So, if you ever find yourself ugly crying after deadlifting, don't sweat it. You're not broken—you're just releasing some deep, pent-up stuff. It's like therapy, except you're squatting your feelings out.

No, You Won't Turn into a Bodybuilder Overnight

Let's bust one of the biggest myths that keeps women from lifting weights: the fear of bulking up overnight like the Hulk. Trust me, if that were possible, I'd already be crushing buildings with my biceps by now. I'm not.

Building muscle takes time, dedication, and effort. Lifting weights won't make you look like Arnold Schwarzenegger, but it will make you feel like a superhero. It's one of the best things you can do for your mind and body, and the confidence that comes with getting stronger? Unmatched.

Cut the Energy-Drainers

Protecting your Fit Babe Energy isn't just about what happens in the gym. It's about cutting out the things—or people—that drain you dry. And let me tell you, that list can get long if you're not paying attention.

Media Detox

One of the first things I did was cut out the news. In 2011, I pulled the plug because the constant doom and gloom? It was draining. The media thrives on negativity, and I didn't want to absorb that anymore. Instead, I filled my brain with things that uplift me—whether it's podcasts, inspiring shows, or books that motivate me.

Toxic Relationships

We're going there—cutting out toxic people. If someone is constantly draining your energy, it's time to set boundaries. You don't owe anyone your emotional energy, especially if they're not adding value to your life.

Your Own Self-Doubt

Your biggest energy drainer? The voice inside your head telling you you're not good enough. I've had to shut that voice down more times than I can count, and every time I do, I get a little of my energy back.

Boundaries, Baby

I learned the hard way that saying "no" is not only okay—it's necessary. I was a people-pleaser for years, always putting others before myself. But you can't pour from an empty cup, and once I started setting boundaries, I felt like I got my life back. Protect your energy, say no when you need to, and stop feeling guilty about it.

Declutter Your Mental Space

Ever notice how Steve Jobs wore the same thing every day? That's because decision fatigue is real. The more choices you make, the more drained you get. I took a page from his book and started simplifying everything. My workout clothes? All the same. One meal a day is always peanut butter on an English muffin. By cutting out those small decisions, I saved my energy for what really matters.

In Conclusion: Guard Your Fit Babe Energy Like Your Life Depends On It

Protecting your energy is everything. The world is full of distractions, toxic people, and energy-draining habits, but when you take control of what you let in, you become unstoppable.

Set boundaries. Simplify your life. Choose what matters, and cut out the rest. When you guard your Fit Babe Energy, you're not just surviving—you're thriving.

Chapter 11

The Fit Babe Workout – My Muscle-Building Secret Sauce (Home Edition)

Let's be real: lifting weights after 40 is a total game-changer. It's not just about building muscle—it's about building confidence, resilience, and strength in every sense of the word.

And the best part? You don't need a gym. All you need is a few pairs of dumbbells, a weight bench (preferably and you can find them on Facebook marketplace all the time) and the commitment to show up for yourself. Because when you're lifting those weights at home, you're not just building your body—you're building your Fit Babe Energy. You're proving to yourself, rep by rep, that you're capable of more than you ever thought possible.

So grab your dumbbells, follow this home workout plan, and get ready to feel stronger, more powerful, and more alive than ever before. Fit Babe Energy is all about showing up for yourself—and trust me, once you start, you'll never look back.

Remember that hilarious return to the gym I talked about? The one where I could barely lift a 10-pound dumbbell and thought I might burst into tears at any moment? Well, I survived. And not only did I survive, but I actually thrived.

Fast forward a few years, and now I've developed a home workout routine specifically designed for women over 40. If I can do it at home, you can too. Here's the thing: lifting weights isn't just about building muscle or looking fit in a bikini (though, let's be real, that's a nice perk). It's about strength—physical, mental, and emotional. It's about showing up for yourself, pushing through the hard stuff, and realizing just how much you're capable of.

Before we dive into the nuts and bolts of my muscle-building secret sauce, let's clear something up: lifting weights will *not* turn you into the female version of Arnold Schwarzenegger. I don't care what anyone says—you're not going to wake up one morning with biceps bigger than your head just because you did a few sets of curls. Building muscle, especially for women over 40, takes time, patience, and yes, some serious effort.

But here's the truth: Your muscles need different things at different ages. When you're under 40, it's all about high reps and light weights to tone and sculpt. After 40? It's about going heavy. And guess what? You can do it all at home with just a few pairs of dumbbells. We're talking dumbbells that make you question your life choices halfway through a set. That's where the magic happens. Your body responds to that kind of challenge by getting stronger. And let's be real—strong is the new sexy.

Cardio Confession: Why I Don't Do It (And Why That's Okay)

Now, here's something that might surprise you: I don't do cardio. Like, at all. And I'm not the only one. After three years on my fitness journey, I've been part of several weight-training groups for women over 40, and guess what? Many of the most badass, inspiring women in those groups say they don't do cardio either.

When someone posts an incredible before-and-after photo and gets asked, "What's your cardio routine?" they often reply, "I don't do any." And let me tell you, the shock is real.

I'm one of those women. And even Jillian, my perfect-bodied trainer, wasn't a fan of cardio. We would do maybe five minutes of warm-up, and that was it.

But here's the thing: after sustaining a few minor injuries early on—always because I hadn't warmed up properly—I realized the importance of warming up your muscles. So yes, I do recommend spending a few minutes warming up and stretching during and after your workouts. Not only does it prevent injuries, but it also feels amazing. Stretching is like the cherry on top of your workout sundae—it helps your muscles recover faster and leaves you feeling good.

That said, I'm still not a fan of intense cardio classes. Those aren't for me. You'll never catch me in a room full of women red-faced and dripping sweat as they push through a class that looks like it could be a military bootcamp. The thing about those classes? They're exhausting, and the benefits are short-lived. You're burning calories in the moment, sure, but as soon as you walk out the door, that's it.

When you build muscle, though? Your body works *for* you 24/7. Muscle burns more calories even when you're not working out. You're building something that keeps on giving. Work smarter, not harder—that's my motto.

How Often Should You Work Out with Weights?

Let's talk about how often you should be working out with weights. The short answer? As often as you can. But before you roll your eyes and think, "Oh great, she wants me to live in the gym," hear me out.

Here's the thing: I'm not a fan of scheduling those mandatory rest days. Why? Because, honestly, your body knows how to recover. It's smarter than we give it credit for. Right now, with my crazy life—juggling kids, work, and trying to remember the last time I did laundry—I'm getting in about five workouts a week, each lasting around an hour. And before you ask, "Are you insane?!" let me clarify. I barely sweat.

Yes, you heard that right—I don't get winded or leave the gym looking like I just ran a marathon through the desert. This isn't cardio boot camp where your goal is to out-sweat the person next to you. Weight training is different. It's about controlled, focused movement. It's about lifting heavy, taking strategic breaks between sets, and feeling powerful without feeling like you're about to pass out in a puddle of sweat. And the best part? The benefits of lifting last way beyond that hour you spend in the gym.

The Magic Formula: Build Muscle, Burn Fat, Rinse, and Repeat

Now, let me lay down a little secret: if you want to transform your body, you've got to build muscle. No, not just for the aesthetics—though trust me, the toned look is a bonus—but because muscle is like your body's secret weapon for burning calories 24/7.

Here's why: cardio burns calories, but only while you're doing it. Once you step off that treadmill, the calorie-burning party comes to a grinding halt. But with muscle? Muscle is like that friend who keeps the party going long after everyone else has gone to bed. The more muscle you have, the more calories you burn around the clock, even when you're binge-watching Netflix or lounging on the couch with a snack.

And if you want to cut fat? Yes, you'll need to be in a calorie deficit—burning more calories than you're eating—but here's the kicker: lifting weights makes that easier. By building muscle, you're turning your body into a calorie-burning machine, so even when you're resting, those muscles are working for you, torching calories like a boss.

Your Body: The Ultimate Art Form

Here's where the fun really starts: lifting weights will become your craft, and your body? It's your art form. You'll learn what works for you and what doesn't. You'll tweak, adjust, experiment, and—just like with any great work of art—sometimes you'll make a masterpiece, and sometimes you'll end up with a blob that looks like it should go back to the drawing board. But every lift, every rep, is a stroke on that canvas.

One thing you'll notice when you start looking at people who are truly in shape—and I'm not talking about "skinny fat" here; I'm talking about strong, lean bodies that look amazing beyond 40—is that they don't have a new workout every week. They're not flipping through the latest fitness trends or hopping on every new YouTube workout video. They stick to a plan and *rinse and repeat.*

Sounds boring, right? Wrong. It's brilliance. It's efficiency. They make a plan, and they work that plan to perfection. There's no need for constant change. Why reinvent the wheel when you've found what works? Stick to the basics, and do them well.

The Power of Push, Pull, Legs (Repeat)

Now, here's my magic formula: push, pull, legs. Simple, right? It's nothing fancy, but it's powerful. Well, actually, I do *push, legs, pull, legs, push, legs*—but you get the idea. You don't need to be doing a thousand different workouts or confusing your muscles with crazy new moves every week. Focus on mastering the fundamentals, and you'll be amazed at the progress you make.

Your body loves consistency, and it rewards you for it. Every time you show up, lift heavier than you think you can, and push your own limits, you're teaching your body to adapt and get stronger. You don't need a million different exercises—just a few that you execute with laser focus and intensity.

You Are Stronger Than You Think—So Push Your Limits

Here's something most people don't realize: you're stronger than you think. Seriously. I can't tell you how many times I've seen women shy away from heavier weights because they're afraid of getting "too bulky" or because they don't believe they're capable of lifting them. Newsflash: you are capable.

Lift heavier than you think you can. Push your own limits. Every time you pick up a weight that scares you just a little bit, you're building strength—not just physical, but mental strength too. You're proving to yourself that you can handle more than you thought possible. And that's where real growth happens.

Lift Heavy, Rest Between Sets, and Watch the Magic Unfold

Let's get real: lifting heavy isn't about flailing through a million reps at lightning speed. It's about control. When you're lifting weights, take your time. Rest between sets, breathe, and recover. You're not here to rush; you're here to sculpt. Weightlifting is a dance—there's rhythm to it, and when you find your flow, it becomes something you actually look forward to. Because nothing feels as good as getting stronger.

Muscle-Building Is Smarter Than Cardio

The beauty of weight training is that it's not about killing yourself with intensity. It's about building something that works for you all day, every day. When you lift weights, your muscles continue to work long after the workout is over. They burn calories even while you're sitting on the couch, sleeping, or scrolling through Instagram. The metabolic benefits of building muscle are huge.

That's why I don't need cardio, and neither do you. (Unless you genuinely enjoy it—then by all means, go for it!) The point is, building muscle gives you long-lasting results. Your muscles become calorie-burning machines, making your body more efficient and helping you stay lean without needing to exhaust yourself.

The Importance of Lifting Heavy After 40

Here's where things get even more important. After the age of 40, muscle mass naturally starts to decline. And as much as we hate to admit it, this decline can lead to all kinds of issues—loss of strength, slower metabolism, increased body fat, and even a higher risk of injury. That's why weight training isn't just a nice-to-have—it's a necessity for women over 40. And science backs this up.

Dr. Stacy Sims, an expert in female physiology and exercise science, has done extensive research on lifting for women over 40. Her work shows that resistance training is one of the most effective ways to combat the natural decline in muscle mass, bone density, and metabolism that happens as we age. According to Dr. Sims, lifting heavy weights helps women maintain muscle mass, improve bone health, and keep their metabolism running efficiently.

She also emphasizes that women in perimenopause and menopause respond better to heavy lifting than to endurance-based exercises. In fact, focusing on lifting heavier weights with fewer repetitions has been shown to significantly improve body composition and strength in women over 40.

My Home Workout Plan: Push, Pull, and Legs

Ready to get started? Let me share my ultimate home workout plan for push, pull, and leg days. This is the exact routine I use to build muscle, strength, and—most importantly—confidence, all without stepping foot in a gym.

Push Day: The Upper Body Powerhouse (At Home)

Push days are all about hitting the chest, shoulders, and triceps. These muscles help you push things—whether that's a door, a shopping cart, or, you know, your kids out the door when you're running late for school drop-off.

But here's the deal with push day: it's not just about pushing. It's about lifting, pressing, and moving weight in a way that makes you feel like a total badass. There's something about pushing heavy weight above your head that instantly makes you feel more powerful, more in control.

Here's how I structure my *at-home* push day:

1. **Dumbbell Bench Press** – 4 sets of 8-12 reps

   Focus: Chest

   We're starting with the big one—the dumbbell bench press. If you don't have a bench, the floor works just fine. Press those dumbbells up, and feel the power in your chest, shoulders, and triceps.

2. **Dumbbell Shoulder Press** – 4 sets of 8-12 reps

Focus: Shoulders

Whether you're sitting or standing, pressing those dumbbells overhead will light up your delts. By the end of this, your arms will feel like they've been through the wringer—in a good way.

3. **Dumbbell Incline Chest Fly (Floor Version)** – 3 sets of 10-12 reps

Focus: Upper Chest

No bench? No problem. Use the floor for your incline chest fly and focus on controlling the movement. It hits your upper chest and makes your favorite V-neck shirt pop.

4. **Dumbbell Lateral Raises** – 3 sets of 12-15 reps

Focus: Shoulders

This is where shoulder sculpting happens. Lateral raises target those side delts. Go slow and controlled—you'll feel the burn in no time.

5. **Dumbbell Skull Crushers** – 3 sets of 10-12 reps

Focus: Triceps

Target the back of your arms with skull crushers. Use your dumbbells and watch those triceps firm up, waving goodbye to any flab.

6. **Dumbbell Front Raises** – 3 sets of 12-15 reps

   Focus: Front Shoulders

   Lift those dumbbells in front of you for a serious front delt workout. These are great for building strength where it counts, especially when you're carrying those heavy groceries.

7. **Push-Ups** – 3 sets of max reps

   Focus: Chest, Triceps

   Push-ups are the ultimate bodyweight exercise. Drop to the floor and see how many you can knock out—you'll be surprised how strong you are.

8. **Dumbbell Overhead Tricep Extensions** – 3 sets of 10-12 reps

   Focus: Triceps

   Finish strong with overhead tricep extensions. This move will round out your push day and leave your arms shaking in the best way possible.

Pull Day: The Back and Biceps Bonanza (At Home)

Pull day is all about the back and biceps—the muscles that help you pull things toward you. And no, you don't need a fancy machine to get this done at home. Just grab those dumbbells and let's go.

Here's the *at-home* breakdown:

1. **Dumbbell Bent Over Rows** – 4 sets of 8-12 reps

   Focus: Back

   Bent over rows are essential for building a strong back. Hinge at the hips, grab your dumbbells, and row like you're pulling something heavy out of the water.

2. **Single-Arm Dumbbell Rows** – 3 sets of 8-12 reps per arm

   Focus: Back

   One arm at a time! Single-arm rows are great for evening out any muscle imbalances. Keep it slow and controlled.

3. **Renegade Rows** – 3 sets of 8-10 reps

   Focus: Back, Core

   Plank position, dumbbell in hand, row to your side. These bad boys hit your back and your core at the same time. Bonus points for keeping your core engaged the whole time.

4. **Dumbbell Reverse Flyes** – 3 sets of 10-12 reps

   Focus: Rear Shoulders

   Reverse flyes hit the rear delts and improve posture. Just because we're working from home doesn't mean we can't walk tall.

5. **Dumbbell Shrugs** – 3 sets of 12-15 reps

   Focus: Traps

   Shrug it out with your dumbbells. This exercise is simple, but it's gold for building those upper back and trap muscles.

6. **Dumbbell Bicep Curls** – 4 sets of 10-12 reps

Focus: Biceps

The classic bicep curl. Squeeze at the top and watch your arms start to take shape.

7. **Dumbbell Hammer Curls** – 3 sets of 10-12 reps

Focus: Biceps, Forearms

Hammer curls are a slight variation that hit both the biceps and forearms. Keep those palms facing inward and curl away.

8. **Dumbbell Concentration Curls** – 3 sets of 10-12 reps

Focus: Biceps

Take a seat, focus on every rep, and squeeze those biceps with concentration curls. It's all about form here.

Leg Day: The Glute-Growing, Quad-Burning Adventure (At Home)

Leg day doesn't require a squat rack or leg press machine to be effective. With just your dumbbells, you can get an amazing lower body workout at home. Your legs are your foundation—strong legs mean strong everything.

Here's my *at-home* leg day:

1. **Dumbbell Squats** – 4 sets of 8-12 reps

   Focus: Quads, Glutes

   Squats are the king of leg exercises. Hold a dumbbell in each hand, squat down, and feel your quads and glutes fire up. Go low and feel the grow.

2. **Dumbbell Romanian Deadlifts (RDLs)** – 4 sets of 8-12 reps

   Focus: Hamstrings, Glutes

   RDLs are perfect for hitting your hamstrings and glutes. Hinge at the hips, keep that back flat, and lower those dumbbells. Your hamstrings will thank you later.

3. **Dumbbell Lunges** – 3 sets of 10-12 reps per leg

   Focus: Quads, Glutes

   Lunges are brutal but effective. Step forward, dumbbells in hand, and watch your legs turn to jelly—in the best way.

4. **Step-Ups with Dumbbells** – 3 sets of 10-12 reps per leg

   Focus: Quads, Glutes

   No fancy step box? Use a sturdy chair or step. Step-ups are fantastic for leg strength and balance.

5. **Dumbbell Goblet Squats** – 3 sets of 10-12 reps

   Focus: Quads, Glutes

   Hold a dumbbell at your chest and squat deep. Goblet squats will light up your quads and glutes.

6. **Dumbbell Glute Bridges** – 3 sets of 10-12 reps

   Focus: Glutes

   Place a dumbbell on your hips and bridge up. Squeeze at the top and feel your glutes working overtime.

7. **Dumbbell Calf Raises** – 4 sets of 15-20 reps

   Focus: Calves

   Don't forget those calves! Stand tall, hold your dumbbells, and raise up onto your toes. Your calves will burn, but it's worth it.

8. **Sumo Squats with Dumbbells** – 3 sets of 10-12 reps

   Focus: Inner Thighs, Glutes

   Take a wide stance and squat down with a dumbbell in your hands. This one targets those hard-to-reach inner thighs and glutes.

Building Muscle After 40: Your Secret Weapon

Lifting weights after 40 is a total game-changer. It's not just about building muscle—it's about building confidence, resilience, and strength in every sense of the word. And the best part? You don't need a gym. All you need is a few pairs of dumbbells, a weight bench, and the commitment to show up for yourself.

Because when you're lifting those weights at home, you're not just building your body—you're building your Fit Babe Energy.

You're proving to yourself, rep by rep, that you're capable of more than you ever thought possible.

So grab your dumbbells, follow this home workout plan, and get ready to feel stronger, more powerful, and more alive than ever before. Fit Babe Energy is all about showing up for yourself—and once you start, you'll never look back.

Chapter 12

Lifting for Libido and Anti-Aging—The Ultimate Double Win Over 40

Alright, buckle up, because we're about to dive into a topic that gets whispered about in late-night texts but is crucial for women over 40: the connection between lifting weights, libido, and anti-aging. And no, this isn't just about getting a firm butt (though, hey, that's a nice perk). We're talking about feeling strong, sexy, and ageless, and how weight training has the power to transform your life from the inside out. If you've ever wondered how to reclaim your confidence in the bedroom and slow down the aging process, guess what? You've hit the jackpot.

Let's start with the elephant in the room: libido. It's something most women are way too shy to talk about, but trust me, we're all thinking it. As we get older, things change. Maybe it's hormones, maybe it's the chaos of life, or maybe it's just the reality of balancing kids, work, and trying to squeeze in some self-care time. Whatever it is, a lot of women find themselves struggling to feel as sexy and connected to their bodies as they once did. And here's the kicker— so much of it has to do with how we feel about ourselves.

Now, I know we're not supposed to compare ourselves to men, but come on, let's do it for a second. Men have no problem going from couch potato to sexy time without so much as a glance in the mirror. Doesn't matter if it's 3 a.m. on a Tuesday or if they've skipped the gym for a month—they're ready. Meanwhile, us? We're over here calculating whether it's the right time of day, how we're feeling about our thighs, and whether the lighting is going to show the stretch marks. It's like we've got this mental checklist that we can't stop obsessing over.

And that, my friends, is why we're in our heads too much.

Why Women Are Stuck in Their Heads

We live in our heads, ladies. We overanalyze, overthink, and second-guess everything from the color of our lipstick to the exact curvature of our hips. We've all been there: a romantic moment is about to happen, and instead of feeling excited, we're stressing about whether we remembered to shave or if our stomach looks bloated. I mean, it's hard to be present when you're busy calculating how much laundry is piling up.

Here's the thing—while we're busy overthinking, most men are just... well, not. They don't care about the dimples on their love handles or the five pounds they gained over the holidays. They're not worried about whether the lighting in the room is flattering. They're just happy to be in the moment, enjoying themselves. And honestly, we should take a cue from that.

But for women, feeling sexy and tapping into our feminine energy often depends on how we feel about ourselves. We need to look good and feel good to fully embrace that nurturing, playful, flirtatious side of ourselves—the side that's been buried under a mountain of self-consciousness and a to-do list the size of Texas. That's where lifting weights comes in and changes the game.

The Confidence-Boosting Power of Weight Training

You see, weight training isn't just about sculpting your body—though that's a fantastic side effect. It's about creating a new relationship with yourself. When you start lifting weights, something magical happens. You begin to see yourself differently. Those moments when you lift a heavier dumbbell than you thought possible, or when your arms start to take on definition, you're like, "Wait a second... is that me?"

And yes, that is you.

When you start feeling stronger, your confidence naturally increases. It's hard to feel self-conscious about your body when you're deadlifting more weight than you ever thought possible. You realize that your body is capable of so much more than you've been giving it credit for. And that confidence? It follows you everywhere. It sneaks into every corner of your life—from the way you walk into a room to the way you feel about yourself in intimate moments.

Feeling strong translates to feeling sexy. When you feel good about your body, you stop nitpicking every little detail, and suddenly, you're present. You're in the moment, enjoying yourself, and guess what? That's when you can truly tap into your feminine energy—your ability to flirt, love, and nurture without a second thought. It's that flow state we're all chasing but can't quite reach when we're too busy overanalyzing ourselves.

Get to Know Your Body—Inside and Out

Let's be honest: most of us don't actually *know* our bodies as well as we think we do. We live with them, sure. We feed them, dress them, even work them out. But when was the last time you really *studied* your body? Not in some "pinch and poke" inspection way, but in a way that feels curious, even a little bit exciting?

We're talking about touching, feeling, *exploring*. Get a mirror, get some time alone, and—yes, I mean it—take a long, delicious look. Trace your collarbone, feel the strength in your arms, and run your fingers over the curve of your hips. God created this beautiful body of yours, and it's yours to know, to learn, to savor. When you start to appreciate your body, not just for what it looks like but for what it feels like, you're unlocking something powerful.

Most women go their whole lives without fully understanding the landscape of their own body. And why? We get so caught up in diets, gym plans, and expectations that we don't slow down to simply *enjoy* ourselves. But that changes today. Today, you're going to become the expert on *you*. You're going to learn every curve, every line, and every place that lights up when you touch it. It's time to explore what feels good and to reclaim your sensuality for yourself.

Teach Your Body's Language

Once you know what makes you feel good, you're ready to teach your partner about your body—about the things that make you feel alive, lit up, and connected. Because here's a little secret: the more confident you are with your own body, the easier it is to *communicate* that to him. No more guessing, no more hoping he'll figure it out. You'll know what you want, and you'll be able to guide him, creating a shared experience that feels both powerful and playful.

This isn't about following a script or sticking to anyone else's idea of sensuality. This is about fully inhabiting your body, about touching your skin and feeling each inch of it come alive. Think of it as a kind of flirtation with yourself, a deep dive into what makes you feel radiant and sexy. This connection isn't just about attraction; it's about *ownership*. And trust me, once you own your own sensuality, the entire world will feel it.

Lifting Weights and Libido: The Science Behind the Magic

Let's break this down on a more scientific level because, yes, there's some serious biology behind why weight training is a game-changer for libido. First of all, lifting weights increases testosterone and growth hormone levels. And before you freak out, I'm not saying you're going to turn into the Hulk. Women naturally have lower levels of testosterone than men, but it's still crucial for our overall health—especially when it comes to sexual desire.

When you lift weights, you're boosting your body's natural production of testosterone, which helps improve libido. It's like your body saying, "Hey, remember me? Let's have some fun." But it's not just hormones—weight training also improves blood flow, which means better circulation, which means, ahem, everything feels a little more alive and sensitive. Wink, wink.

There's another layer to this: endorphins. Lifting weights releases those feel-good chemicals that not only help reduce stress but also make you feel more connected to your body. That post-workout glow? It's not just about sweating out toxins; it's about feeling empowered and in control of your physical self. And trust me, when you feel in control of your body, your mind follows suit.

Aging Gracefully (And Strongly)

Now, let's switch gears and talk about the ultimate anti-aging hack: lifting weights. I know, I know, we've all heard the same tired advice about how "age is just a number" and "you're only as old as you feel." But let's be real for a second. As women, once we hit 40, things start to shift. Hormones fluctuate, metabolism slows down, and suddenly, the things that used to work for us—like eating a bagel for breakfast without gaining five pounds—just don't cut it anymore.

Enter: weight training. Lifting weights after 40 is like discovering the fountain of youth, but without the cheesy, too-good-to-be-true promises. Here's what happens when you start lifting: you build lean muscle mass, and lean muscle is the secret sauce to staying youthful. It helps to rev up your metabolism, burn fat more efficiently, and keep your body strong and toned. And let's not forget, it's also a key player in maintaining bone density.

You want to avoid the "shrinking as we age" phenomenon? Lift weights. Strong muscles support strong bones. In fact, studies have shown that resistance training helps prevent osteoporosis, which is a big deal as we get older. Your future self will thank you for building that strength now.

The Fountain of Youth Is Made of Dumbbells

Here's another fun fact about aging—skin elasticity, the thing that keeps us looking youthful, starts to decline as we get older. But guess what helps? Lifting weights. By improving circulation and stimulating muscle growth, strength training can help improve your skin's firmness and elasticity. It's like turning back the clock without any invasive procedures.

Now, let me be clear: lifting weights isn't going to erase every line or wrinkle, but it will keep you feeling youthful, energetic, and strong. You'll move better, feel more vibrant, and have the kind of energy that's rare for women over 40. It's about aging gracefully and powerfully. You're not just fighting the effects of aging—you're thriving through them.

How It All Connects: Libido, Anti-Aging, and Feeling Amazing at Every Age

Lifting weights is the ultimate win-win. It boosts your libido, helps you age gracefully, and most importantly, it makes you feel damn good about yourself. When you look in the mirror and see those muscles forming, when you feel strong enough to lift things you never thought possible, it transforms not just your body, but your mind.

Weight training is about empowerment. It's about stepping into the best version of yourself—one who is confident, strong, sexy, and unapologetically feminine. It's not about fitting into someone else's idea of beauty or femininity. It's about defining your own.

The Takeaway

Here's the bottom line: If you want to boost your libido, age like a queen, and tap into your true feminine power, start lifting weights. It's not just about getting fit; it's about reclaiming your confidence, your energy, and your life. You deserve to feel amazing at every age, and lifting weights is one of the best ways to get there.

So, pick up those dumbbells, embrace the process, and let's redefine what it means to feel strong, sexy, and ageless. Your body—and your confidence—will thank you.

Chapter 13

Fit Babe Energy in Everyday Life

You know how they say, "What happens in the gym, stays in the gym"? Yeah, that's not true at all. At least not when it comes to Fit Babe Energy. The best part of tapping into this mindset isn't just that you can crush a set of squats or finally see some definition in your biceps. Nope. It's that this energy, this confidence, this strength—it spills over into every part of your life.

Fit Babe Energy doesn't just live in the dumbbells and deadlifts. It goes beyond the gym and starts to show up in places you didn't even realize needed a little extra muscle. It's how you walk into a room with your head held high, even when you're the only person there who doesn't have a clue what's going on. It's how you handle a tough day when everything is falling apart, but you know—deep down—that you're going to get through it, because you've lifted heavier things before (including your own self-doubt).

In this chapter, we're going to talk about what happens when you take Fit Babe Energy out of the squat rack and into the rest of your life. It changes everything. And the best part? It's funny, it's empowering, and yes, you'll feel like a badass.

How Confidence Impacts Every Area of Your Life (Yes, Even That Awkward Parent-Teacher Conference)

Let me start by telling you something that might sound obvious but is easy to forget: confidence is contagious. And I don't mean the kind of confidence you fake when you're trying to impress someone. I'm talking about the kind of confidence that comes from showing up for yourself day in and day out. The kind that's built from pushing through those last few reps when you thought you couldn't, and from keeping promises to yourself, even when it would've been easier to hit snooze.

When you have that kind of confidence, it follows you everywhere.

Take work, for example. Pre-Fit Babe Energy, I used to walk into meetings hoping no one would ask me hard questions. I'd sit there, nodding along, secretly praying the attention stayed far away. But after I started lifting weights, something shifted. It wasn't that I suddenly knew all the answers or magically became the smartest person in the room. It was just that I felt... stronger.

Lifting heavy things makes you realize that you can handle heavy stuff—physically and mentally. It's like, "Okay, I survived a brutal leg day yesterday, and I'm still standing. So what if they ask me a tough question? I got this." That strength? It trickles into your work life, your relationships, and even the way you parent your kids.

Speaking of parenting—let's talk about how Fit Babe Energy shows up when you're dealing with a toddler tantrum in the middle of Target. Before Fit Babe Energy, I might have felt my patience wearing thin. But now? Oh, now I know I've got this. Why? Because if I can handle three sets of Romanian deadlifts, I can handle this meltdown with grace. (And maybe a little bribery. I mean, I'm not a saint.)

The thing is, confidence—real, earned confidence—makes you a better parent, a better partner, and honestly, a better human. When you feel good about yourself, it radiates. People pick up on that energy. It's not about being cocky or arrogant; it's about having a quiet, steady belief in yourself that comes from knowing you've put in the work.

Why You Need to Celebrate Every Win, No Matter How Small

One of the biggest lessons I've learned on this journey is the importance of celebrating every win—and I mean every single one. You nailed your workout today? Celebrate it. You made it through a tough day without losing your cool? Celebrate it. You resisted the urge to eat an entire sleeve of Oreos? Celebrate it (maybe with just one Oreo).

We're so conditioned to think that only the big wins count. You know, the huge milestones like losing 20 pounds, hitting a new personal record in the gym, or finally getting that promotion. But what about the little victories? The ones that, when stacked together, are what actually get you to those big milestones?

I used to be the type of person who would blow past my small wins without even acknowledging them. I'd finish a workout, feel good for about five seconds, and then immediately start thinking about what I needed to do next. But that's not how Fit Babe Energy works.

Fit Babe Energy is about recognizing that progress is progress, no matter how small. It's about celebrating the fact that you showed up today, even if you weren't feeling it. It's about giving yourself a pat on the back for sticking to your goals, even when the world was trying to throw you off track.

One of the best ways to do this? Track your wins. Keep a journal, or use the notes app on your phone, and write down something you're proud of every day. It doesn't have to be earth-shattering. Maybe you finally nailed that tricky yoga pose, or maybe you managed to squeeze in a workout before the kids woke up. Whatever it is, celebrate it. Because the more you celebrate your wins, the more wins you'll start to see.

How to Attract the Life You Want by Embracing Your Inner Fit Babe

Here's where things get a little woo-woo, but stick with me. I'm not saying that lifting weights will suddenly make all your dreams come true (although, wouldn't that be nice?). But there is something to be said for the idea that what you put out into the world, you get back.

When you embrace your inner Fit Babe—when you carry that energy with you—you start attracting things that align with that energy. It's not magic; it's mindset. You start seeing opportunities where you used to see obstacles. You start believing in your ability to achieve your goals, and that belief drives your actions.

For example, I used to shy away from challenges. If something felt too hard or too risky, I'd convince myself it wasn't for me. But after I started lifting and building that Fit Babe Energy, something shifted. I started going after things I wanted. I applied for opportunities I would've been too scared to try for before. I took risks in my business, in my personal life, and guess what? A lot of those risks paid off.

That's the thing about Fit Babe Energy—it's not just about how strong you are physically. It's about how strong you are mentally. When you start showing up for yourself, when you start keeping promises to yourself, it creates momentum. And that momentum? It attracts more good things into your life.

But here's the catch: you have to be open to it. You have to believe that you're worthy of the life you want. It's not enough to just lift weights and hope for the best. You have to take that energy and apply it to everything you do.

Fit Babe Energy in Relationships (AKA, How to Raise Your Standards Without Guilt)

Fit Babe Energy doesn't just transform your body or mindset—it shifts how you approach your relationships too. When you start showing up for yourself, respecting your own boundaries, and embracing your worth, it naturally changes how others respond to you. You set the tone for how you expect to be treated, and suddenly, the dynamics in your relationships begin to evolve—sometimes in ways you didn't anticipate.

It's not about blaming anyone else or playing the victim; it's about recognizing where you've been putting yourself last, often unintentionally. For years, I'd catch myself trying to keep everyone around me happy—whether it was at work, with friends, or in my personal life. It wasn't about resentment or sacrifice, but more a pattern of putting my own needs on the back burner. But as I leaned into Fit Babe Energy, I began to see that part of growing stronger is learning how to prioritize yourself, unapologetically.

This wasn't about demanding more from others—it was about expecting more from myself, first. I started to see that healthy boundaries were necessary, not as a way to push people away, but as a way to create space for the right kind of energy to flow into my life. It wasn't always easy, and not everyone embraced the changes, but I knew this wasn't about pleasing others. It was about aligning my relationships with the life I wanted to build.

Romantic relationships were no different. I used to think that certain compromises or behaviors were just part of the deal. But once I fully embraced where I wanted my life to go, it became clear that I deeply desired a partnership where both people showed up for each other fully, where respect and support were mutual. It wasn't about rejecting others—it was about choosing to live in a way that honored who I was becoming, and knowing that the right future relationships would rise to meet me.

Fit Babe Energy and Parenting: Raising Strong, Confident Kids

Let me tell you something about parenting: your kids are watching. Every time you handle a challenge, every time you talk about yourself, and every time you show up in the world, they're absorbing it. You might think they're too busy with their screens to notice, but trust me—they notice everything.

When I started embracing Fit Babe Energy, I saw a shift not just in myself but in how I was raising my kids. Suddenly, the lessons weren't just about them; they were about me too. I realized I needed to stop being so hard on myself. No more striving for the mythical mental model of Supermom, because frankly, she doesn't exist (and if she does, she's probably exhausted). It wasn't just about raising strong, confident kids anymore—it was about showing them how to bounce back, handle life's curveballs, and get back up after falling down.

The Shift in Parenting: Showing, Not Telling

As I started regulating my own energy, I realized how important it was for my kids to see that taking care of yourself isn't selfish—it's essential. They saw me set boundaries, say "no" to things that didn't serve me, and prioritize my mental and physical health. And you know what? They started doing the same. Watching them take ownership of their own well-being made me prouder than any A+ report card ever could.

I stopped trying to be the do-it-all-mom—the one who never makes mistakes and always has everything under control. Instead, I showed my kids that it's okay to fail. It's okay to have off days, it's ok to be completely wrong, and it's ok to say I am sorry. What matters is how you handle it and how you get back up.

Fit Babe Energy: The Gift You Give Your Kids

Here's the thing about Fit Babe Energy: it's contagious. When you start living with intention, confidence, and resilience, your kids soak that up. You're not just telling them to be strong—you're showing them what that looks like in real life.

I'm not saying I've got it all figured out. Some days, I'm still a mess. But I've learned that my energy matters—not just for me, but for my kids. By taking care of myself, I'm giving them permission to take care of themselves too. And that's the real win.

Fit Babe Energy in Everyday Life: Conclusion

Fit Babe Energy doesn't stop at the gym door. It's everything. It's how you approach your entire life. It's about discipline at the smallest level—those tiny promises you keep with yourself that compound into something much bigger. When you carry that energy into your work, relationships, and daily routine, everything shifts. You become the kind of person who doesn't just dream big—you make things happen.

So here's my challenge: take that Fit Babe Energy with you everywhere. That discipline, belief, and determination? It's the key to unlocking everything you want. Fit Babe Energy is your life, and there's no ceiling on what you can achieve.

Chapter 14

Start Where You Are – Ready or Not

Let me tell you something nobody really talks about when it comes to fitness, life changes, or, well, any kind of transformation: you're never going to feel ready. Not fully. Not completely. There will never be this perfect, magical moment where the stars align, your schedule clears up, and you suddenly feel like Beyoncé in her prime. Trust me—I waited for that moment, and you know: it never showed up.

So, here's the thing: you don't need to wait. In fact, you *shouldn't* wait. Start before you're ready, right where you are. Because the truth is, you'll never feel ready, but you can absolutely start anyway.

I Wasn't Ready, But I Jumped In Anyway

Let me take you back to the beginning of my journey. I wasn't exactly in top form. My stomach had been through three pregnancies, my abs were torn apart, my body was tired, and I was juggling more than I thought I could handle. I wasn't ready to start this whole fitness journey. Not even close. I had a laundry list of reasons why I should wait: my stomach wasn't lean enough, I wasn't strong enough, I didn't have the time, I wasn't "there" yet.

But one day, I decided to jump in anyway. I told myself, "If I wait until I'm 'ready,' I'll never start." That's a fact.

Was I in perfect shape? Absolutely not. Am I in perfect shape now? Nope. But here's the kicker: I'm on the journey. And that's what matters. Because waiting for perfection, or waiting for some ideal version of yourself to show up, is just an excuse to avoid doing the hard stuff.

We all have this fantasy version of ourselves in our heads, right? You know, the version who has the perfect abs, never skips a workout, and walks around looking like a fitness model. I call her "Future Me," and she's always doing things way better than Present Me. But here's the problem: Future Me doesn't exist until Present Me starts doing the work. That leaner, fitter version of me that I was waiting for? She wasn't going to show up unless I started showing up first.

The Myth of "Being Ready"

Here's another thing I've learned along the way: the idea of "being ready" is a myth. It's something we tell ourselves to delay the discomfort of starting. It's like saying, "I'll start running once I'm fit," or "I'll go to the gym when I'm stronger." It's backward thinking because getting fit or stronger is the result of starting, not the prerequisite.

And listen, I get it. Starting is scary. It's uncomfortable. It's so much easier to wait until you feel more confident, more prepared, more "ready." But here's the truth: *ready never comes*. You're always going to find something that makes you feel like you're not quite there yet.

I didn't think I was ready to help others either. In fact, I almost didn't start this entire fitness journey because I told myself, "Who am I to inspire other women when my stomach isn't as lean as I want it to be?" I wanted to wait until I had the "perfect" body, until I looked like the women I followed on Instagram. But guess what? Those women aren't real life, and waiting to be perfect is just another excuse.

Jump in and Get Started

One of the most powerful lessons I've learned is that you don't have to be ready to start—you just have to *start*. Perfection is a trap, and waiting for it will keep you stuck in the same place for years.

When I finally stopped waiting and started showing up for myself, I realized that progress happens in the doing, not in the waiting. It wasn't about waiting until my stomach was leaner or until I had more time in my day. It was about getting up and doing the work, even when I didn't feel like it, even when I didn't feel ready.

And you know what? The most amazing things started to happen once I let go of the idea of "ready." I began to build strength. I started seeing changes—not just in my body, but in my mindset. I stopped being so hard on myself. I started celebrating small wins. I showed up at the gym, not because I was ready, but because I was committed.

Start Before You're Ready, Because You'll Never Be Ready

Here's something I want you to take away from this chapter: start now. Not tomorrow, not next week, not when you've lost 10 pounds, or when your schedule clears up. Start now, because you'll never feel fully ready. You'll never reach that perfect moment when everything falls into place. Life doesn't work like that.

And here's the thing—once you start, you'll realize that you didn't need to be ready. You just needed to begin. The confidence, the strength, the results—they come from doing the work. Not from waiting for the perfect conditions.

I hear this all the time from women who say, "I'll start working out when I'm in better shape," or "I'll join the gym once I lose a little weight." But the gym is where you get in better shape. Lifting weights is how you build strength. You don't need to be anything other than who you are right now to start.

The same goes for anything in life—whether it's starting a new job, going back to school, or deciding to make a major life change. Waiting for the "perfect" time is just fear dressed up as procrastination. And guess what? You can move forward even when you're scared.

Imperfect Action Beats Perfect Inaction

Let me give you another gem of wisdom: *imperfect action beats perfect inaction every single time.* It doesn't matter if you don't have the perfect workout routine or the perfect diet plan. It doesn't matter if you're still figuring it all out as you go. What matters is that you're doing *something*.

When I first started lifting weights, I didn't know what I was doing half the time. I wasn't sure if I was doing the exercises correctly, I didn't know which foods would fuel my body the best, and I certainly didn't feel like I was in the best shape of my life. But I kept going. I kept showing up. And those small, imperfect actions added up.

The same goes for helping others. I wasn't ready to become someone who could inspire other women. I didn't feel like I had all the answers, and I wasn't the picture of perfection I thought I needed to be. But I realized something important: you don't have to be perfect to make an impact. You just have to be honest and authentic. And sometimes, that's more powerful than perfection.

The Journey Is the Destination

Here's the truth about transformation: there's no final destination. There's no moment where you suddenly arrive and say, "Well, I'm done now! I've reached the end of the journey." The journey *is* the destination. It's about who you become along the way, not just what you achieve.

If I had waited until I was "ready," I wouldn't be here now, writing this book. I wouldn't have started lifting weights, I wouldn't have started sharing my journey, and I definitely wouldn't have started helping other women find their own strength. But because I decided to start before I was ready, I've been able to experience this incredible transformation—and help others do the same.

So, I'm here to tell you: start now. Don't wait until your body is perfect, or your schedule is clear, or your confidence is sky-high. Jump in right where you are, with all your imperfections, and get started. Because the longer you wait, the longer it will take to see the changes you want.

You're Ready Now

Here's the big secret: you're already ready. You might not feel like it, but you are. Everything you need to get started is already inside you. You don't need a perfect body, or a perfect plan, or perfect timing. You just need to believe in yourself enough to take that first step.

And once you do? Everything changes. You'll start to see that the fear, the doubt, the excuses—they were just distractions. You'll realize that you're stronger than you thought, braver than you gave yourself credit for, and more capable than you ever imagined.

The Lies We Tell Ourselves to Stay Comfortable

Here's the thing: it's easy to stay in your comfort zone. The lie we tell ourselves is that comfort is safe. But here's a secret: *comfort zones are where growth goes to die.* They're the cozy little nests we build for ourselves, where everything feels familiar and easy. But they're also the places where we stagnate, where we convince ourselves that we're not ready, or that we'll start "tomorrow." You know what happens in comfort zones? Not much.

Staying where you are might feel safe, but it's also keeping you stuck. We use the "I'm not ready" excuse because it's easier than admitting we're scared of the unknown. We fear failure, we fear judgment, and we fear the discomfort that comes with growth. But here's what I've learned: growth happens when you push through the fear. It's in those moments when you're uncomfortable and unsure that real transformation begins.

And let me tell you—it's worth it. Every uncomfortable step forward is one step closer to the person you're meant to be.

Imperfection Is Your Superpower

There's this false idea floating around that everything has to be perfect before you can start. It's like we've convinced ourselves that if we're not 100% prepared, if we don't have the perfect plan or the perfect body or the perfect circumstances, then we shouldn't even bother. But let me tell you: imperfection is your superpower.

When you start messy, when you start before you're ready, you're giving yourself permission to be human. You're giving yourself space to grow, to learn, and to figure it out as you go. And guess what? That's where the magic happens. It's not in the perfect execution—it's in the willingness to show up, to make mistakes, and to keep going anyway.

So embrace the mess. Embrace the fact that you don't have it all figured out. None of us do! But the difference between those who move forward and those who stay stuck is the willingness to act despite the uncertainty.

In Conclusion: Jump In, Messy and Unready, and Just Start

Perfection is the enemy of progress. Waiting for the right time is the quickest way to stay stuck. So, do yourself a favor—start now. Start where you are. It won't be perfect, but it will be real, and it will be yours.

I didn't think I was ready to transform my body, and I certainly didn't think I was ready to help others do the same. But I jumped in anyway, and I'm so glad I did. Because that leap—the one you take when you're scared, unprepared, and not quite ready? That's where the magic happens.

Fit Babe Energy isn't about waiting until you're perfect. It's about showing up, doing the work, and trusting that you'll get stronger along the way. You're not waiting for your best self to arrive—you're becoming her with every single step forward.

Now, it's your turn. Jump in. Get started. You're more ready than you think.

Chapter 15

The Joy of Doing Hard Things (And Yes, It's Supposed to Suck at First)

Alright, let's get real for a second—doing hard things is like waking up on a Monday with no coffee in the house. It sucks. But here's the kicker: it's *supposed to* suck. That's what separates the goal-getters from the ones who daydream about them. The magic of change isn't in the beginning where everything feels like you're trying to bench press a rhinoceros—it's in what comes after. It gets easier. A lot easier.

And before you think I'm spouting motivational fluff, let me hit you with some science. Behavioral experts have done the work, and they all say the same thing: the hardest part isn't actually the hard thing itself. Nope. The hardest part is deciding to *start*. Once you've made that decision, your brain does a little happy dance and says, "Fine, let's do this." Then things start to shift. This is what researchers call the "three-phase model of behavior change," but I like to call it "The Oh-No-I-Started-This-Thing-And-Now-I-Have-To-Keep-Going Plan."

Phase One: The 'I've Decided, So I Guess I Have to Do This Now' Moment

Making the decision to do something hard is like standing on the edge of a cliff, looking down, and thinking, *"This might be a horrible idea."* Your brain? It's screaming, *"Retreat! Get back to your comfort zone! There's pizza there!"* But once you leap—once you say, "Alright, let's do this"—everything shifts.

For me, it was deciding to go back to the gym after an embarrassing four-month hiatus. Now, mind you, before that, I was feeling like a certified badass. I had been working with Jillian, my trainer, lifting weights, feeling strong, and then...BOOM! December happened. The holidays, colds, and excuses started flying faster than I could stop them.

The old me would've thrown in the towel, set up shop on the couch with Netflix, and justified every reason to stay there. "You missed too much time," "You'll never get back to where you were," "There's a new season of *Bake Off,* why go to the gym?" But here's the deal—those thoughts are just your brain's sneaky way of trying to keep you safe in your cozy little bubble. Don't fall for it.

Phase Two: Actually Showing Up—AKA the Struggle Bus

Now that you've made the decision to start, you've gotta actually...show up. And let me tell you, that first day back in the gym felt like someone had swapped out my weights for small cars. My muscles? MIA. My confidence? Somewhere under the gym mat. It was like being in one of those dreams where you show up to school in your underwear, only it was worse because I was wearing workout gear that I no longer deserved to wear.

But showing up? That's the hardest part. It's the mental barrier that says, *"You don't belong here anymore,"* but you do. The first day might feel like you're dragging yourself through quicksand, but that's just the warm-up. What you're really doing is planting a big ol' flag that says, *"I'm here, and I'm not going anywhere."*

Phase Three: Muscle Memory—Your New Best Friend

Here's where the magic happens. Scientists (aka super-smart people with clipboards) call it "neuroplasticity," but let's just call it "getting your groove back." After a few weeks of consistent effort, your brain and body stop fighting you and start adapting. This is where muscle memory kicks in.

Even though it felt like I had lost every ounce of strength during my gym hiatus, my body remembered. And that's the beauty of it—once you start working those muscles, they're like, *"Oh yeah, we've done this before!"* Within a few weeks, the weights didn't feel so heavy anymore, and my form came back. I wasn't starting from scratch; I was just waking up the dormant badassery that had been taking a nap.

Lean Into the Discomfort, Baby!

Let me tell you something: the discomfort you feel at the beginning? That's the secret sauce. When you lean into the hard stuff, that's where the magic happens. You're breaking through the walls that have been holding you back, and it's in those moments when you want to quit that you start discovering your real strength.

It sounds twisted, but doing hard things actually becomes addictive. No, really. Once you start experiencing the high that comes from pushing through the struggle, you'll find yourself seeking out new challenges. Suddenly, the impossible starts feeling possible. Heck, it starts feeling *fun*.

I know, I know—fun? Hard things? Who am I kidding? But trust me, the first time you tackle something that felt insurmountable and come out the other side, you'll be like, "What else can I conquer?"

Beware the Comfort Zone—It's a Trap!

Here's where I need to throw up a warning sign: comfort zones are sneaky little traps. They lull you into a false sense of security, telling you that staying put is good enough. But here's the deal—nothing grows in the comfort zone except your Netflix queue and possibly your waistband.

Growth only happens when you push beyond what feels safe. The more you step out of your comfort zone, the easier it becomes. And that's when you start realizing you're capable of a whole lot more than you ever gave yourself credit for.

The Power of Doing Hard Things in Everyday Life

Now, let me take a moment to show you how doing hard things applies to literally everything else in life. It's not just about deadlifts and squats—this mindset creeps into all the corners of your life. Take parenting, for example. (Yes, parenting is a hard thing, and yes, it's supposed to suck at first, too.)

You ever try to get three kids out the door on time while also attempting to drink a cup of coffee and remember that, yes, it's picture day, so no, they cannot wear their dinosaur PJs to school? Hard. But guess what? The more you do it, the more you realize you can handle the chaos. Just like lifting weights, it gets easier with time (though no promises about that dinosaur PJ thing).

Or how about your career? Let's be real—work isn't all sunshine and promotions. You're going to have days where everything feels like it's crashing down, where deadlines are looming, and you're one awkward Zoom call away from calling it quits. But just like in the gym, showing up, doing the hard thing, and pushing through that discomfort is where real growth happens. You don't hit PRs (personal records) in your career by staying in your comfort zone. You get there by taking on the tough projects, asking for the raise, and yes, sometimes failing along the way.

When Life Punches You in the Face—You Get Back Up

Let me hit you with another truth bomb: Life's going to knock you down. It's inevitable. Maybe you'll miss a workout. Maybe you'll fall off the meal plan. Maybe the universe will throw something massive at you that you weren't expecting. But here's the thing: it's not about the fall—it's about how fast you get back up.

I could've easily let those four months of gym absence turn into forever. But instead, I decided to show up, do the hard thing, and push forward. And because of that, I came out stronger. That's the beauty of doing hard things—you get knocked down, but when you get back up, you're more powerful than before.

This mindset applies to everything: fitness, relationships, career, and even self-care. Doing hard things teaches you resilience. It shows you that setbacks aren't permanent, and that failure is just part of the process. The more you practice getting back up, the better you get at it. And trust me, *you will get knocked down.* But the next time life punches you in the face, you'll know exactly how to throw a right hook back.

The Science of Sucking (at First)

Let's circle back to the science behind why doing hard things sucks at first. Your brain is literally wired to avoid discomfort. It's like, *"Why would I willingly put myself through something hard when I could just...not?"* Your brain wants to keep you safe, and by "safe," it means stuck in the same old routine.

But here's the beauty of it: the more you push yourself out of your comfort zone, the more your brain adapts. It's called neuroplasticity, which is just a fancy word for saying your brain is capable of rewiring itself. When you do something hard—whether it's lifting weights, running that first mile, or tackling a new project at work—you're creating new neural pathways. Over time, the hard thing becomes easier, and your brain starts to crave that challenge.

Think of it like leveling up in a video game. The first level is tough because you're figuring everything out, but by the time you're on level 10, you're a pro. Your brain works the same way. Each time you do something hard, you're leveling up your resilience, your strength, and your ability to handle whatever life throws at you.

Embrace the Suck—It's Where Growth Lives

Here's what I want you to remember: doing hard things is supposed to suck at first. That's the whole point. If it were easy, everyone would do it, and it wouldn't be special. The fact that it's hard is what makes it transformative. It's where growth lives.

So the next time you find yourself struggling—whether it's in the gym, at work, or in life—don't shy away from the discomfort. Lean into it. Embrace it. Because on the other side of that struggle is where you find your strength.

Conclusion: Go Do the Hard Things (Yes, You)

Let me sum it up for you: Doing hard things is the secret sauce to leveling up in life. Yes, it's uncomfortable. Yes, it's challenging. But it's also the most rewarding thing you'll ever do. And here's the kicker—once you make the decision to start, everything else falls into place. It won't be easy, but it will be worth it.

It's not about being perfect. It's about showing up every day and doing the work. It's about leaning into the discomfort and realizing that's where the growth happens. So go ahead—embrace the suck, do the hard things, and watch how your life transforms. Because once you start, there's no stopping you.

Chapter 16

The Promise I Made to You
(And to Myself)

Let's rewind for a second. Remember that Facebook post I made? The one where I said, "Hey world, I'm gonna get my life together, and maybe we can do it together"? I didn't know it then, but that post was a line in the sand. It was like saying, "I'm doing this—no backing out now." It was a promise, not just to myself, but to you. And like all good promises, it came with the fine print: "Yes, this is going to get messy, chaotic, and downright ridiculous at times."

I promised to share the whole journey—the ugly, sweaty, tear-filled parts—and not just the glossy "after" picture. Why? Because we both know life isn't some perfectly curated Instagram feed. Transformation doesn't come with filters. It's more like trying to put together IKEA furniture without the instructions.

So here we are, at the end of the book, but let's be real—this isn't the end of anything. This is just the beginning. This chapter, my dear reader, is a reminder. A reminder that transformation isn't about perfection. It's not about getting everything right the first time or even the tenth time. It's about showing up, day after day, doing the work, and trusting the process. And if you're reading this, I've got good news—you're already on the right path.

Fit Babe Energy: The Journey of Becoming

Fit Babe Energy is for the woman who thought she was broken, for the mom who looked in the mirror and said, "Who is this tired stranger?" It's for the woman who's over 40 and has been told her best days are behind her (pfft, yeah right). It's for anyone who's been stuck in the same cycle, trying to make a change and ending up at square one with a tub of ice cream and Netflix asking, "Are you still watching?"

I see you. I was you.

But let's set the record straight: you're not broken. You never were. You're stronger than you think, more powerful than you realize, and your best days? Oh honey, they aren't behind you. They're standing right in front of you, waving like a crazy person, waiting for you to show up.

Let me say that again for the people in the back: your best days are right in front of you. Not in some distant memory of what you used to be, but right here, right now. And the way you get there? By showing up for yourself. Embrace your Fit Babe Energy. Own it. Believe that you are worth the effort it takes to transform. That's the key—it's not about becoming someone else, it's about becoming the most kickass version of yourself.

The Secret Sauce: It's Time to Own Your Fit Babe Energy

Here's the thing: Fit Babe Energy is what's going to take you from "I can't" to "Wait, I just did that." It's the belief that you are worth the time, the energy, and the effort to show up for yourself. It's like a secret superpower that you didn't know you had, just waiting to be unlocked.

When I started on this journey, I didn't believe I was worth it. I thought I was too far gone, too tired, too... you know, mom-ish. But guess what? I was wrong. And if you're sitting there thinking the same thing, you're wrong too.

You're not too far gone. You're not too old. You're not broken. You are exactly where you need to be to start right now. But there's a catch (there's always a catch, right?): You have to own it.

It's not about waiting for the universe to hand you an invitation. It's about believing that you're capable of more than you ever thought possible. And once you start showing up for yourself, trust me— doors will start opening. And I'm not just talking about gym doors. I mean all the doors: the ones that lead to better relationships, better health, better careers—better everything.

Owning Your Fit Babe Energy: It's Not About Perfection

Now, let's be clear: this isn't about being perfect. Fit Babe Energy doesn't require you to get it right every time. There are going to be days when you eat pizza instead of salad (and you should—pizza is practically a love language). There will be mornings when you hit snooze five times. It's fine. You're human. Fit Babe Energy isn't about perfection—it's about persistence.

It's about getting back up after you fall, brushing the crumbs off your shirt, and showing up again. It's about realizing that just because you stumbled doesn't mean you failed. It means you're in the game. And as long as you keep showing up, you're winning.

The Promise I Made to Myself (And to You)

When I made that Facebook post, I didn't know what kind of crazy rollercoaster I was signing up for. I didn't know how many times I'd feel like throwing in the towel or how many meltdowns I'd have mid-burpee. But I made a promise—to myself and to you—that I would keep showing up. And here I am, holding up my end of the bargain.

That promise wasn't about abs or jeans sizes (although, let's be real, fitting into your favorite jeans feels amazing). It was about proving to myself that I could do hard things. That I could transform, not just my body, but my mindset, my relationships, my entire life. And that's the promise I made to you: You can do hard things too.

Fit Babe Energy: The Transformation Beyond Fitness

Here's what I want you to take away from all of this: Fit Babe Energy isn't just about fitness. It's about transforming the way you think about yourself and the way you show up in the world. It's about believing that you are worth every ounce of effort it takes to become the best version of you.

This isn't about abs—it's about becoming a woman who believes in herself, even when the odds are stacked against her. It's about knowing that no matter how many times you fall, you can (and will) get back up. It's about realizing that you have the power to change your life, and no one can take that away from you.

Your Best Days Are Right in Front of You

If you take away just one thing from this book, let it be this: Your best days are right in front of you. I don't care if you're 25 or 55, if you've been stuck in a rut for years, or if you've tried and failed more times than you can count. You are capable of more than you think.

There's no perfect moment to start. There's just now. And the truth is, your best days are the ones where you show up for yourself, where you push through the hard stuff, where you choose to keep going even when every part of you is saying, "Nah, I'm good."

The Future Is Yours—Now Let's Get Started

So here we are. The end of the book, but not the end of the journey. Fit Babe Energy isn't just something you carry with you to the gym—it's something you carry with you everywhere. It's the thing that's going to help you tackle every challenge, overcome every setback, and open doors you never thought possible.

My advice? Don't wait. Don't wait for Monday, don't wait for January, and don't wait for some magical "right moment." Start right now, today, with whatever you've got. Because here's the thing—when you embrace Fit Babe Energy, when you own it, when you show up day after day, you'll look back and realize that the best part wasn't reaching the goal. The best part was becoming the woman who got there.

I'd Love to Hear from You!

Your journey matters, and I'd love to hear all about it. If you're on this fitness journey, or even just thinking about starting, find me on Instagram at **@finding_fearless** and let's connect! Share your wins, your struggles, and everything in between.

And if you're curious about Sweet Minerals makeup and want to try out **The Flawless Face**, here's a special gift for you—**use coupon code 40PLUSFITFRIEND** at checkout on sweetminerals.com for 20% off, just for being a reader of this book.

Keep pushing, keep shining, and keep owning your Fit Babe Energy! You've got this. 💪